Accelerating CNS
Drug Development

This book is dedicated to our patients, their families, and their caregivers. Special thanks to Maria Elena Weiss for her constant inspiration.

Accelerating CNS Drug Development

NEAL R. CUTLER, M.D.
JOHN J. SRAMEK, PHARM.D.
California Clinical Trials, Beverly Hills, California, USA
NEIL M. KURTZ, M.D.
MICHAEL F. MURPHY, M.D., PH.D.
and
ANGELICO CARTA, M.D.
Worldwide Clinical Trials, Atlanta, Georgia, USA and London, UK.

JOHN WILEY & SONS
Chichester · New York · Weinheim · Brisbane · Singapore · Toronto

Other Wiley Editorial Offices

John Wiley & Sons, Inc., 605 Third Avenue,
New York, NY 10158-0012, USA

WILEY-VCH Verlag GmbH, Pappelallee 3,
D-69469 Weinheim, Germany

Jacaranda Wiley Ltd, 33 Park Road, Milton,
Queensland 4064, Australia

John Wiley & Sons (Asia) Pte Ltd, 2 Clementi Loop #02-01,
Jin Xing Distripark, Singapore 129809

John Wiley & Sons (Canada) Ltd, 22 Worcester Road,
Rexdale, Ontario M9W 1L1, Canada

British Library Cataloguing in Publication Data

A catalogue record for this book is available from the British Library

ISBN 0-471-98128-1

Printed from camera-ready copy supplied by the authors
Printed and bound in Great Britain by Biddles Ltd, Guildford and King's Lynn
This book is printed on acid-free paper responsibly manufactured from sustainable forestry, in which at least two trees are planted for each one used for paper production.

Contents

Foreword

The development of drugs designed to treat CNS disorders presents some of the most difficult challenges in any area of pharmaceutical research. Such complex human illnesses as psychosis, depression, anxiety, or dementia can never be reflected accurately by animal models, and clinical endpoints in these conditions are not readily defined with objectivity and precision. The added pharmacokinetic problems posed by the blood/brain barrier make it especially difficult to predict effective clinical doses. It is not surprising that some 8–12 years of a new product's patent life are used in research and development, and the motivation to improve on this is clearly high.

The authors have a unique track record in the development of CNS drugs—their collective experience being far greater than that of any individual pharmaceutical company. In this book, they have distilled this knowledge into a valuable and practical guide covering the common problems associated with CNS drugs. These include the selection of the right clinical dose, the most suitable target patient population, and the optimum study design, controls, and endpoints. I found their review of how animal data can be best extrapolated to humans and the strengths and weaknesses of 'animal models' in predicting clinical efficacy particularly valuable. There is also excellent coverage of clinical trial design options and surrogate biochemical, physiological, and endocrine endpoints that are increasingly important in providing objective measures of the effectiveness of CNS drugs. Perhaps the greatest strength and originality in the authors' approach concerns their advocacy of 'bridging studies' to assist in the choice of clinical doses for CNS drugs. Such clinical studies are conducted at the end of Phase I or early in Phase II in patients rather than in healthy volunteers, and are designed with an escalating dose regimen to identify the 'minimum intolerated dose'—which yields unacceptable adverse effects—the dose below this determining the 'maximum tolerated dose' (MTD). Their experience with this approach has shown firstly that patients suffering from CNS illnesses (Alzheimer's disease, schizophrenia, depression, or anxiety disorders) surprisingly often tolerate significantly higher doses of CNS agents than healthy control subjects, and secondly that the clinical MTD is clearly of key importance in the design of the optimum clinical trial for any CNS drug—ideally, this should be combined with knowledge of the corresponding pharmacokinetic and pharmacodynamic parameters. The discussion of bridging studies is enriched with many individual examples from recent CNS drug development research.

The present volume comes at a particularly timely moment as new moves to streamline the FDA regulatory process are under active consideration in the United

States, and it represents an excellent addition to the literature in this field and will
surely be widely read.

Leslie L. Iversen, Ph.D., F.R.S.
Department of Pharmacology
University of Oxford, U.K.

ACKNOWLEDGEMENT

We would like to thank Janis Schaap for her valuable assistance in preparing this book; also to Wanda Krall, Ph.D., Julie Smutko Daugherty, and Paul Smith for their technical help.

Also of interest to readers:

Optimizing the Development of Antipsychotic Drugs
J.J. Sramek, N.R. Cutler, N.M. Kurtz, M.F.Murphy and A. Carta
0471 97011 5   1997

Anxiolytic Compounds
Perspectives in Drug Development
N.R. Cutler, J.J. Sramek and N.M. Kurtz
0471 95713 5   1996

Pharmacodynamics and Drug Development
Perspectives in Clinical Pharmacology
Edited by N.R. Cutler, J.J. Sramek and P.K. Narang
0471 95052 1   1994

Alzheimer's Disease
Clinical and Treatment Perspectives
Edited by N.R. Cutler, C.G. Gottfries and K. Siegfried
0471 95039 4   1994

Alzheimer's Disease
Optimizing Drug Development Strategies
N.R. Cutler, J.J. Sramek and A.E. Veroff
0471 95145 5   1994

1   Introduction

WHY DO WE WANT TO ACCELERATE DEVELOPMENT?

The development of new drugs in the United States presents an interesting dilemma. While the demand for newer and better compounds is seemingly insatiable, public concern over the safety and effectiveness of these compounds has prompted some of the most stringent regulatory requirements in the world. Thus, investigators must complete increasingly extensive preclinical and clinical testing programs, which can translate into substantial development timelines. As the economic burden of disease has been estimated at $400 billion dollars annually in the United States alone, there is a significant motivation to accelerate the development of safer and more effective compounds.

Unfortunately, drug development is itself an expensive venture, and only a small fraction of the compounds that undergo the initial phases of testing will ever gain the approval of the Food and Drug Administration (FDA). The average cost of development for a new chemical entity (NCE) has been estimated at $350 million (Stave and Joines, 1997), and the time span from synthesis to marketing approval nearly 12 years (DiMasi et al., 1991). Research and development (R&D) expenditures by U.S. pharmaceutical companies alone have risen from $10.9 billion in 1992 to $15 billion in 1996 (Stave and Joines, 1997).

The emphasis on novel strategies to treat CNS disorders and the reduced role of me-too drugs have contributed to the increase in R&D costs. Many of the advances in disease treatment are due to research conducted by the pharmaceutical industry, which often reaches far beyond the development of a single new drug. Indeed, Kaitin et al. (1993) noted that of the 196 NCEs approved by the FDA from 1981 through 1990, 92% had their source in the pharmaceutical industry. However, although pharmaceutical R&D has led to significant progress in understanding disease mechanisms, as well as provided innovative new compounds for their treatment, drug companies have increasingly been forced to defend their R&D activities (and expenses) to society (McKercher, 1992).

Rising R&D costs are coupled with a short patent life of new compounds, providing additional motivation to accelerate the development process. Although the General Agreement on Tariffs and Trades (GATT) treaty has extended the patent life to 20 years, the first 8–12 years of patent coverage are generally spent in R&D (Stave and Joines, 1997). This combination of increased R&D costs and the short timeframe for a product to realize a return on its investments often translates into higher product prices for the consumer, leading to threats of pharmaceutical pricing regulations by the government (DiMasi, 1994; FDC Pink Sheet, 1993). This prospect, in turn, has raised arguments from pharmaceutical companies that controlled drug prices could stall research progress (American Journal of Hospital Pharmacy News, 1994). Meanwhile, the changing marketplace with the growth of managed care has already begun to exert effects upon pharmaceutical sales.

The high cost of drug development is also due to the high scientific standards which a drug development program must meet prior to approval in the United States. There are several stages of development which a new compound must complete successfully in order to gain marketing approval. Prior to testing in humans, a preclinical program assessing both the toxicology and pharmacology of the compound is required. The main purpose of the preclinical program is to provide a rationale, resolve formulation issues, describe biodisposition, and identify potential toxicities in humans, so that these events can be anticipated and monitored in later clinical trials. The assessment of several species, at least one rodent and one non-rodent, is often included in order to yield as much information as possible that could be useful in human testing. Additionally, if animal models are available which are thought to be predictive of efficacy for that particular indication, the compound may be subjected to this kind of testing (this subject is discussed in more detail in Chapter 2).

A clinical development program includes a series of studies to assess a compound's safety and efficacy (the phases of clinical development are discussed in more detail in Chapter 5). Initially, single doses of the compound are administered to small numbers of healthy subjects in a carefully monitored setting. Often the doses for these studies are based upon safety information gleaned from preclinical testing. If the initial studies indicate that the compound is well tolerated, the safety of multiple doses is then tested in larger groups of subjects. If the compound continues to be well tolerated, studies will be performed to assess its safety and tolerability in patients with the target indication.

Once a safe and tolerable dose range has been identified in the target population, the efficacy of the compound is investigated. Since the Kefauver-Harris amendments were passed by Congress in 1962, new compounds must demonstrate not only safety, but also substantial evidence of efficacy prior to marketing approval. To achieve such evidence, well-designed, randomized controlled trials have become the cornerstone of a drug development program. Alternative paradigms are also useful at this stage for further scientific and medical product profiling. The investigational compound is tested in increasing numbers of patients, eventually culminating in large, definitive (or 'pivotal') efficacy trials. The goal of these trials is to find 'substantial evidence' that the drug will have the effects it claims, defined as:

> evidence consisting of adequate and well controlled investigations, including clinical investigations,... on the basis of which it could fairly and responsibly be concluded... that the drug will have the effects it purports to...have...

Currently, the regulatory requirements have included at least two adequate and well-controlled clinical trials for CNS compounds. The request for a minimum of two trials is in line with the scientific principle of replication (Katz, 1993); however, one large study may be acceptable in non-CNS indications. These trials are time-consuming and account for a large percentage of the total R & D costs, but they are necessary in order to meet the scientific standards of the industry as well as the safety and efficacy demands of the consumer.

Finally, if there is convincing evidence that the compound is clinically effective, large-scale, open trials are conducted in order to assess its safety and efficacy in a more representative sample of the population in which the drug will be marketed. The issue of generalizability is always a significant factor, as patients in clinical trials may not be representative of the general patient population. While the clinical development program is being carried out, additional animal studies are also conducted to assess the long-term toxicological effects of the compound.

Thus, the design of each study in a development program is based in large part upon information acquired in previous studies. Without careful planning at each stage, incomplete or inaccurate results of one study can lead to larger problems in later development. Problems during any of the above stages can be extremely costly, and can delay or even halt a drug development program.

WHAT CAUSES DEVELOPMENT TO STAGGER?

There are several elements which contribute to a well-designed and efficient clinical trial. Likewise, there are several areas in which lack of planning can cause a program to falter. The literature has outlined several potential problems in the clinical trial process (Klein, 1991; Katz, 1993) which can result in costly delays, or even the discontinuation of a drug development program (Box 1.1). While this list is far from complete, it highlights some of the most common pitfalls in clinical drug development.

Moreover, there are several potential problems specific to the development of new drugs for CNS disorders. Psychiatric patient populations are often quite heterogeneous, which can lead to significant variability in a given sample despite rigorous diagnostic algorithms. Increased variability can, in turn, lead to ambiguous or misleading results. For example, schizophrenic patients can vary widely in terms of positive and negative symptoms, and acute or chronic status of their illness. Additionally, efficacy studies of CNS drugs rely upon clinical rating scales that can be subjective and unreliable, without assiduous attention to the details of execution. In studies which lead to critical go/no-go decisions, problems with inter-rater reliability or high placebo effects can seriously affect a drug development program. Thus, careful, well-designed and executed trials are necessary to help researchers avoid these problems, and to complete the requirements of a CNS drug development program in a timely manner.

BOX 1.1 COMMON PROBLEMS IN CLINICAL DRUG DEVELOPMENT

Inaccurate dose selection
Poor selection of target population by inexperienced clinicians
Poor protocol
Incorrect length of study period
Unrepresentative sampling with high attrition rates
Lack of appropriate control group
Inappropriate or unspecified endpoint measures
Inappropriate or unspecified statistical analysis
Statistical analysis based on detecting statistical rather than clinical significance

---

Dose Selection

Inaccurate dose selection is a good example of how a lack of planning in one area can cause an entire development program to stagger. The importance of proper dose determination for clinical testing is recognized in the scientific literature (Turri and Sten, 1986; Schmidt, 1988; Katz, 1993) as well as the FDA guidelines on the clinical evaluation of drugs. The probability of detecting therapeutic benefit and avoiding potentially serious adverse events is dependent on the selection of an optimal dose range for efficacy studies.

In order to make informed decisions about dose selection, detailed data about the tolerability of the compound is required. One problem that can occur early in clinical development is a failure to identify the maximum tolerated dose (MTD). As Katz (1993) has noted, the FDA is 'aware of many examples where no systematic attempt has been made to achieve this level, with the result that potentially testable (and perhaps more effective) doses are never incorporated into efficacy trials.' Schmidt (1988) also observed that inadequate doses are often chosen in an effort to avoid attrition in later studies, and that the goal is 'to use the minimum effective dose rather than the optimal one.' For the majority of CNS compounds, therapeutic efficacy tends to increase with increasing dose; thus, a failure to evaluate the high end of the tolerated dose range could result in a failure to detect efficacy.

Traditionally, initial safety and tolerability studies of CNS compounds are conducted in healthy volunteers. Consequently, even if an MTD is determined, differences in tolerance between patients and healthy subjects can lead to inaccurate dose selection. Such differences have been noted for nearly every major CNS drug class, including antipsychotics, Alzheimer's disease compounds, antidepressants, and anxiolytics (Miller et al., 1993; Sramek et al., 1995; Grof, 1993; Sramek et al., 1996). In most cases, patients can tolerate higher doses of these compounds than their healthy counterparts. Thus, the tolerable dose range could be underestimated if the MTD is not determined in the target population.

The selection of a dose interval that is too low could cause a development program to be discontinued for lack of efficacy, despite the potential for higher doses to show therapeutic benefit. Alternatively, if a dose range is too high, a development program could also be discontinued due to unacceptable toxicity. In both of these cases, the dose levels could be adjusted after the initial studies; however, this situation would result in costly delays that might have been avoided.

Regulatory Issues

Concern over the time necessary to complete a drug development program is not limited to the pharmaceutical industry. Over the past decade, regulatory agencies have also focused their attention on potential ways in which to accelerate drug development and approval. This focus is partly in response to patient advocacy groups who have questioned whether the time it takes to move a compound through the required stages of development is truly necessary or efficient.

In recent years, increased public and governmental awareness of this issue has resulted in several steps to help expedite the review process. For example, the establishment of prescription drug user fees to help underwrite the cost of hiring additional reviewers has helped the FDA to relieve its backlog of applications and to speed the review of new applications. Most recently, the Senate approved legislation to accelerate the FDA approval of new drugs and medical devices. Among other items, this bill would give the FDA more flexibility in the number of clinical trials deemed necessary to demonstrate the efficacy of new compounds, as well as require the FDA to develop a plan by the year 2000 for clearing its backlog of products awaiting approval.

However, although this legislation could substantially reduce the time required for drug approval, it does not diminish the importance of well-designed trials and conclusive data. A balance must be maintained between the innovation of better CNS compounds and the need to keep a tight regulatory reign on safety.

Learning and Confirming Cycles of Drug Development

Sheiner (1997) has stressed the need for more informative and efficient clinical trials in his recommendation that a process of learning and confirming be applied to drug development. In the context of clinical trials, he suggests that two major learn-confirm cycles should be recognized. The first cycle includes learning what dose of the compound is tolerated in normal subjects and confirming that this dose has the promise of efficacy in a selected group of patients. This cycle culminates in a decision of whether or not to continue the development of the compound. The second cycle includes learning how to use the drug in representative patients to optimize the risk/benefit ratio and confirming that the drug has achieved an acceptable risk/benefit ratio in these patients. If all of these goals are accomplished, approval is granted.

Although learning and confirming studies are necessarily sequential, and can be time-consuming, the information they provide can have potential savings overall in both cost and time. As Sheiner (1997) points out, nothing is as expensive as a failed study late in development. As discussed earlier, there are many ways in which a lack of information can cause a drug development program to falter. Learning trials can provide valuable information that could contribute to more informative trials later in development. Although not all of the questions listed in Box 1.2 require an answer prior to an NDA application, any information that can be gleaned from early clinical studies could contribute to the compound's later success.

Another advantage of learning trials is the assurance that an adequate profile of the drug will be available after approval and marketing. A thorough investigation of the drug's properties can help clinicians to avoid a regimen that could produce serious toxicity, which can result in a loss of market share or even withdrawal. Sheiner (1997) cites the example of midazolam, which was initially marketed at an excessive dose due to a lack of information on its pharmacokinetic/pharmacodynamic profile.

The opportunity to streamline drug discovery and development has the potential to benefit both the pharmaceutical industry and the consumer. However, we do not suggest that streamlining means cutting corners. Careful planning is necessary at every step, from initial preclinical toxicology to large, pivotal efficacy studies. Only through the careful construction of a solid foundation of studies can we hope to conduct well-designed, accurate, and accelerated drug development programs.

BOX 1.2 PRACTICAL QUESTIONS ON THE CLINICAL USE
OF A NEW DRUG

What is an appropriate initial dose for a particular patient?
How soon will the intended effect start?
How long will the intended effect last?
Will tolerance develop?
What happens if the patient misses doses?
What are the chances that the initial dose will require alteration?
What are the indications that a dose requires alteration?
How should the dose be altered? When should it be altered? Should the change
   be made in large or small increments?

Adapted from Sheiner (1997)

REFERENCES

American Journal of Hospital Pharmacy. Drug price controls will cripple research and development, pharmaceutical executives tell Congress [news]. *Am J Hosp Pharm* 1994; **51**(9): 1132.

DiMasi JA. Risks, regulation, and rewards in new drug development in the United States. *Reg Toxicol Pharmacol* 1994; **19**: 228–235.

DiMasi JA, Grabowski HG, Lasagna L. Cost of innovation in the pharmaceutical industry. *J Health Econ* 1991; **10**: 107–142.

FDC Reports Pink Sheet. Breakthrough drug price provisions in Clinton plan are 'modest,' Pryor claims: briefing for Congressional colleagues attempts to cut off expected criticisms. *FDC Reports Pink Sheet* 1993; Oct 4; **55**: 4–6.

Grof P, Akhter MI, Campbell M. *Clinical Evaluation of Psychotropic Drugs for Psychiatric Disorders: Principles and Proposed Guidelines.* Seattle: Hogrefe & Huber, 1993.

Kaitin KI, Bryant NR, Lasagna L. The role of the research-based pharmaceutical industry in medical progress in the United States. *J Clin Pharmacol* 1993; **33**(5): 412–417.

Katz R. The domestic drug regulatory process: why time is of the essence. *Epilepsy Res Suppl* 1993; **10**: 91–106.

Klein DF. Improvement of phase III psychotropic drug trials by intensive phase II work. *Neuropsychopharmacology* 1991; **4**(4): 251–271.

McKercher PL. Issues in health policy: pharmaceutical research and development. *Clin Ther* 1992; **14**(5): 760–764.

Miller AL, Maas JW, Contreras S, Seleshi E, True JE, Bowden C, Castiglioni J. Acute effects of neuroleptics on unmedicated schizophrenic patients and controls. *Biol Psychiatry* 1993; **34**: 178–187.

Schmidt R. Dose-finding studies in clinical drug development. *Eur J Clin Pharmacol* 1988; **34**: 15–19.

Sheiner LB. Learning versus confirming in clinical drug development. *Clin Pharm Ther* 1997; **61**(3): 275–291.

Sramek JJ, Fresquet A, Marion-Landais G, Hourani J, Jhee SS, Martinez L, Jensen CM, Bolles K, Carrington AT, Cutler NR. Establishing the maximum tolerated dose of lesopitron in patients with generalized anxiety disorder: a bridging study. *J Clin Psychopharmacol* 1996; **16**(6): 454–458.

Sramek JJ, Hurley DJ, Wardle TS, Satterwhite JH, Hourani J, Dies F, Cutler, NR. The safety and tolerance of xanomeline tartrate in patients with Alzheimer's disease. *J Clin Pharmacol* 1995; **35**(8): 800–806.

Stave GM, Joines R. An overview of the pharmaceutical industry. *Occup Med* 1997; **12**(1): 1–4.

Turri M, Stein G. The determination of practically useful doses of new drugs: some methodological considerations. *Stat Med* 1986; **5**: 449–457.

2 Antecedents to Clinical Exposure

"Considering possible pharmacokinetic and pharmacodynamic species differences, extrapolation of drug efficacy and toxicity from animals to humans is extremely complicated and difficult, if not impossible. In addition to the relationship between drug concentration and intensity of pharmacological effect, many relevant variables—such as formation of pharmacologically active or toxic metabolites, environmental factors and underlying diseases—must also be taken into consideration."   (Lin, 1995)

In this chapter we consider animal models for the pharmacokinetics, pharmacodynamics, toxicity, and efficacy of novel compounds. Although there are simply too many variables for animal data to be accurately extrapolated to humans, preclinical studies provide an important preview of what may be expected when a drug is tested in humans. Since drug response in animals almost always contains elements that are similar to human response, along with elements that are different, preclinical studies can rarely be used to make quantitative predictions of complex processes but can be extremely useful in suggesting areas that should clinically investigated. The proper interpretation of preclinical results demands skill; the primary utility lies in being able to plan clinical trials that will assess potential outcomes rather than in being able to predict the exact nature of those outcomes.

ANIMAL MODELS AND TOXICITY: APPLICATIONS IN CNS DRUG DEVELOPMENT

The use of animal models to gauge toxicity prior to administration in humans is not exclusive to CNS drugs, nor is the process highly tailored for this class of drugs. There are a few issues unique to CNS drugs which are important to note; we have tried to cover these below. In addition, we will discuss the basic principles of toxicity testing in animal models, giving examples of applications in the development of CNS drugs.

Regulatory Requirements of Toxicity Testing

Toxicity testing is a pivotal aspect of the preclinical regulatory requirements surrounding new drug development. Agencies look to preclinical data to provide animal and in vitro studies of 1) acute, subacute and chronic toxicity tests; 2) tests of the drug's effects on reproduction and the developing fetus; 3) any special toxicity test related to the drug's particular mode of administration or conditions of use; and 4) any in vitro studies intended to evaluate drug toxicity (21 CFR 1.312, 1992).

To date, the most universally accepted guidelines are those published by the Organization for Economic Cooperation and Development (OECD) (Auletta, 1995). There are basic rules relating the animal exposure required before human studies can be conducted. Table 2.1 enumerates some of the minimum requirements (Cereghino and Kupferberg, 1993; Scales and Mahoney, 1991; Alder and Zbinden, 1988). In the conduct of toxicity studies designed to follow regulatory requirements, valuable pharmacokinetic and pharmacodynamic information can also be gained and used to extrapolate from animals to humans. This will be discussed later in more detail.

In 1996, a significant proposal to change toxicology requirements was advanced by Monro and Mehta who suggested that single doses might be safely administered to humans earlier in the development process than was accepted at that time. Their proposal was based on the point that many more drugs are halted in development due to lack of efficacy or adequate pharmacokinetic data in man, rather than adverse events; and at that, adverse events were seldom life-threatening -- particularly in single dose situations where drug accumulation is not an issue. The Center for Drug Evaluation and Research (CDER) responded first in the same publication (Choudary et al, 1996), and later with official guidelines (Guidelines, 1996)

Table 2.1 Minimum animal exposure required prior to human dosing

Human Dosing	Animal Exposure Required*
1 dose	14 days dosing
10 days dosing	30 days dosing
6 months dosing	1 year dosing
1 dose study (multiple volunteers)	14-30 days dosing, 3 doses, subacute toxicity for 2 species, mutagenicity testing
multiple dose study (7-10 days)	30 days dosing, subacute toxicity for 2 species
clinical trials up to 6 months	1 year dosing, chronic toxicity for 2 species, carcinogenicty for 2 species, further mutagenicity, reproduction toxicity

 * intravenously and intended route of administration

wherein single dosing in man might be performed when sufficient acute toxicity data was available from animal models. This has profound implications for CNS drug development, given the historically challenging issue of pharmacokinetics for this class.

Basic Toxicology Designs

In the drug development process, toxicity testing in animals includes acute, subchronic and chronic toxicity evaluations: the distinction between which is duration of exposure (Auletta, 1995). Range finding studies might also be conducted under the auspices of toxicology, however, many of the key elements for determining optimal dose in humans can be collected during studies like the former.

Animal toxicology study designs share a few fundamental aspects. Whether a classical design or newer animal-saving methods is employed, investigators should administer experimental drugs via the same route in animals as the intended route in humans whenever possible. An appropriate number of animals and dose groups should be utilized to provide a basis for risk assessment (International Conference on Harmonization, 1995).

Adverse event profiling begins early in the development process, in hopes that animal response may provide insight into human response. Thus, animals are closely monitored for any observable effects to the animals' health and outward behavior. Necropsy is also conducted to determine cellular-level toxicity in various organ systems, and sometimes to ascertain absorption, delivery, metabolism, and excretion (ADME) information in cases where these cannot or may not be determined during dosing.

Animal toxicity tests are also an integral component in the determination of appropriate human dosing. Estimation of the median lethal dose (LD_{50}) has long been the cornerstone of toxicity testing in animal models. This is the dose at which half of the animals exposed to drug die, and has influenced a variety of analyses to identify appropriate human dosing. Auletta (1995) also describes the median effective dose (ED_{50}), or dose at which half of the animals exhibit an effect of the drug; the no observed effect level (NOEL); the no observed adverse effect level (NOAEL), the no toxic effect level (NTEL), the maximum tolerated dose (MTD), and highest tested dose (HTD). Identifying all of these markers is not usually incorporated into a single toxicity study design, but the compilation of data from the combination of preclinical animal toxicity studies required by regulatory agencies lays the foundation for extrapolating to man. The NTEL or NOAEL dose, measured in several species, is important in determining doses to be administered to man, as will be discussed shortly.

As toxicity testing is, by design, very broad, there are few distinctions in the development of CNS drugs which are worth noting. Perhaps the most significant, however, would be recognizing the ability of CNS drugs to cross the blood brain barrier, thus closer examination of CSF and brain tissue samples may be recommended.

Reducing Animal Subjects

Siglin and Rutledge (1995) define alternative animal models as "any technique that reduces or eliminates the need for live animals and thereby prevents potential pain and distress in animals." Many factors, but especially the reduction of animal suffering, motivate the trend for reducing or eliminating the number of animals used in all stages of medical research.

One fixed dose alternative method was first proposed in 1987 (van den Heuvel et al, 1987) and realized through an international collaborative study (van den Heuvel et al, 1990) wherein smaller groups of animals are dosed simultaneously, as compared with the classical LD_{50} test. Similarly, Bruce (1985; 1987) designed the "up-and-down" method, dosing animals one at a time and adjusting subsequent subject's doses up or down according to reaction to the experimental compound. In a comparison with classical LD_{50} testing (Yam et al, 1991) these two alternative animal models demonstrated good agreement with the classical method, significantly reduced the number of animals required, and provided adequate information to rank test substances according to the EC classification system for acute oral toxicity. This study also found the up-and-down to be the preferred alternative method for approximating lethal dose – an important element in traditional pharmaceutical research – while using the fewest number of animals among the three methods.

Future Trends: *In Vitro* Screening

A future alternative to *in vivo* animal models may be the expanded use of *in vitro* animal models. The last decade has produced greater understanding of drug metabolizing enzymes (Guengerich, 1992; Gonzalez FJ, 1992), and their roles in drug toxification and detoxification (Tephley and Burchell, 1990; Nelson and Harvison, 1987). Thus, species-specific metabolism and toxicology from *in vitro* evaluations can be used increasingly to advance drug development in a more humane and less costly fashion.

Ball et al (1995) divide in vitro studies into the categories of validated screens, valued-added screens, and ad-hoc mechanistic screens. The first of these involves drugs whose mechanisms are well understood and standardized, so confidence in the predictive powers of validated screens is adequate for making critical development decisions. For example, genotoxicity studies, if not species-specific to humans for ethical reasons, must give thorough explanations of mechanism to satisfy regulatory requirements. As research yields greater understanding of mechanisms earlier in development, this category of *in vitro* screening may phase out some early *in vivo* animal testing.

Next, the more broad, value-added screens (for drugs whose mechanism are less well understood) are more likely to accompany *in vivo* screens than replace them. However, value-added in vitro studies with human tissue can be an important resource for ranking relative toxicities, assessing the relevance of animal studies in human therapeutic use, and help to determine the most appropriate species for preclinical studies. Thus, this type of in vitro screen has special application in extrapolating from animal to humans, and is further discussed later in this section.

Lastly, ad-hoc screens are designed to directly study the mechanisms by which drugs cause cellular damage. While this type of screen will never replace in vivo models, they can help investigators to understand the factors which predispose a population or species to toxicity, possibly define mechanisms for detoxification, and thereby streamline the selection process and design for animal models in later development.

Ball et al, (1995) among others (Frazier, 1991) recognize that replacement of in vivo models can only be achieved through extensive validation of in vitro models, and the development of more predictive approaches, such as may be available through the development of mathematical models linking kinetics and dynamics.

Extrapolating from Animals to Humans: Toxicity and Dose

A great deal has been learned by comparing human response to approved or nearly-approved drugs with that of animal models. However, the inaccessibility of late stage human study results for many compounds naturally precludes a better understanding of the pharmacological relationships between humans and animals *during development*. Proceeding down this blind alley requires a great deal of "guess work" in extrapolating data from animals to humans. While there is general agreement that there are more advantages than disadvantages in using animal data to predict risk in humans (Maloney, 1993), fortunately there is a growing number of resources which improve researchers' abilities to anticipate the effects likely to occur in man, and to determine doses which may be safe and perhaps efficacious in first-in-man studies.

Some rudimentary models for determining appropriate dose for humans use linear extrapolation from animal data based on body weight. Body weight *can* be consistently predictive of liver weight, water intake, creatinine clearance, total nitrogen output, hemoglobin synthesis and other parameters (Krasovskij, 1976) across a wide range of species (Calabrese, 1983). However, physiological and metabolic processes such as renal function, metabolic rate and cardiac function are not directly proportional to weight (Voisin et al, 1990) so, though common practice (PDR, 1997), dose extrapolation based on body weight is not optimal.

A slightly more reliable method of dose extrapolation is body surface area, particularly respecting toxicity. Freireich et al (1966) established that, relative to humans, the surface area of mice is roughly 1/12, of rats is 1/7, of monkeys is 1/3, and of dogs is 1/2 the surface area of humans; doses can be estimated accordingly. Unfortunately, not all types of toxicity correlate well with surface area; skin toxicity correlates poorly, and CNS toxicity and peripheral neuropathy -- our area of focus -- deviate considerably from good correlation. There is also the consideration that ADME factors can vary widely, independent of animal size. Sometimes these factors can be explored in value-added *in vitro* studies. Houston (1994) proposed and tested a four stage strategy involving *in vitro* clearance determinations as scaling factors which can be extrapolated with good correlation to *in vivo* models. This use of an *in vitro* study bridges the gap between traditional *in vitro* studies and animal models by narrowing the dosing window, but still does not circumvent the need for preclinical pharmacokinetic studies. Thus, pharmaocokinetic studies in animals are the preferred resource for determining first-in-man dosing and are discussed in detail later in this chapter. At this time, though, it is important to note that their contribution to extrapolating dose from animal to human studies is, in many cases, critical.

Having discussed the measures which are key to extrapolating dose (LD_{50}, ED_{50}, NOED, NOAEL, MTD), and the potential means through which a mathematical extraction might be made (body weight, surface area, pharmacokinetic parameters), let us turn to specific models for honing in on the ideal first-in-human dose which have demonstrated success. In each of these methods, *overestimating* toxicity is favored over underestimating toxicity as the potential adverse outcomes are delayed development versus risk to volunteers.

In the 1950's, the 100-fold safety factor was introduced by Lehmann of the FDA. (Maloney, 1993). Using this method, the investigator first determines a threshold dose level, beyond which a substance causes adverse events in animals. This is equivalent to what we have now termed the NTEL. This dose is divided by ten, based on the assumption that some humans might have greater sensitivity to the experimental compound than do animals. This smaller dose is again divided by 10 to account for variability in sensitivity *among* humans. The resulting $1/100^{th}$ of the NTEL dose in animals is considered, according to this method, an acceptable exposure level for humans.

This principle of the 100-fold safety factor is still used today, although calculations have become more sophisticated. For example, Ford (Cutler et al, 1997) reports that a common practice of extrapolating doses is to determine 1/10 or 1/100 of the NOAEL and multiply that dose by an allometric scaling factor (Voisin et al, 1990). Ascending the dose beyond that point can be undertaken rather aggressively, but this method gives the investigator a reliably safe starting point. Ford notes that often CNS drugs cannot be elevated as rapidly as drugs for other indications. Rather than doubling and doubling again, as some indications allow, drugs for CNS indications are typically raised by the amount of the original dose only (i.e., 1, 2, 3, 4 times the original dose instead of 1, 2, 4, 16 times).

A software program, *Tox_Risk*, has been developed for the unique purpose of extrapolating dose between species, with focus on the issue of human risk (Crouch, 1989). *Tox_Risk* also fits various dose-response curves to the end-of-experiment results of bioassays. Ten different dose-response formulae are utilized by the program in order to produce the maximum estimated likelihood for dose-associated risks, and confidence limits. Factors from animal models such as breathing rate, food and water consumption, body weight, and lifespan are entered, along with drug exposure, to provide appropriate dose either between animal species or from animal to human models.

Extrapolating between animal models and humans for assessing adverse event profiles is a much less straight forward process (Spilker, 1991). Litchfield (1962) found that for six study compounds, 68% of the toxic effects observed in *both* rats and dogs were found in humans and 79% of the toxic effects observed in *either* species were found in humans. Heywood (1984) found extremely poor correlation between rat and dog models and humans. Among 13 adverse events observed in humans from 14 different study compounds, only 7 were observed in animal testing. Johnsson et al (1984) explained that it is difficult to relate human adverse reactions to animal data due to the subjectivity of many of these reactions in humans (such as dizziness, headache, nausea), the fact that doses are often excessive in animals, and immunological effects are difficult to detect in animals. It can be concluded that while we depend on animal models to give us insight regarding potential adverse events, they cannot be heavily relied on to anticipate human response.

Applications in CNS Drug Development

Some examples of using animal data to predict human toxicity for CNS compounds are given below.

Anxiety

A central acting anxiolytic agent underwent various toxicity testing in mice, rats, rabbits, and dogs. In addition to single-dose studies, several multiple-dose study designs were conducted; important findings were that a) a 52-week study of rats found 12.5 mg/kg to be free from toxicological effects; and b) a 52-week study of dogs found 2.5 mg/kg to be free from adverse side-effects. Adverse effects in animals were related to the pharmacological activity of the drug, namely those of the central nervous system. In healthy volunteers, several safety/tolerance study designs were implemented, with doses equating to .0028 to .57 mg/kg, based on a standard of average humans weighing 68 kg. With respect to the 100-fold safety factor method, this dose range represents roughly 1/1000th to 1/5th of the NOAEL found in dogs (the most sensitive species for this compound). Resulting adverse events were mostly related to the central nervous system. On introduction to the target population, doses of more than twice those given to healthy volunteers were given and well tolerated. The MTD in patients with anxiety was identified as 100 mg/day – equating to just over half of the NOAEL in dogs.

Alzheimer's Disease

An acetylcholinesterase inhibitor recently under clinical investigation by the authors has an interesting development history. Preclinical studies in several animal models determined tolerability to this compound to be highly species-specific, thus extrapolation from animal models to humans was not easily accomplished. Adverse effects observed in these models were indicative of excessive cholinergic stimulation and included salivation, lacrimation, loose stools, diarrhea, emesis and convulsions. The NTEL was established as 0.36 mg/kg/day in dogs – the species thought to correlate best with humans. Accordingly, first-in-human doses were very low and safe. Phase II and III trials proceeded at low doses, but efficacy was only marginal. Dosing was then re-examined in the target patient population, and confidently raised to nearly twice that used in the first course of studies, and development of this compound is resuming at this safe and much more efficacious level. Thus, the top dose in man was defined by the NOAEL dose in animals. Although twice this dose was well tolerated in man, it is likely that higher doses could have been well tolerated also.

Schizophrenia

An atypical antipsychotic agent currently under development demonstrated adverse effects in animal models which were related to the pharmacologic activity of the substance and included reduced motor activity, ataxia, and ptosis. Doses on the order of 8-10 mg/kg/day were well tolerated (NOAEL), and non-lethal up to 100 times this range. First-in-man single doses ranged from 1 to 160 mg, and resulting adverse events included dizziness, somnolence, postural hypotension, headache, asthenia and nausea. However, no dose-response relationship was established for adverse events, and no MTD was reached. A bridging study in the target population (patients with schizophrenia) found the drug to be well tolerated in doses up to 300 mg BID, close to the NOAEL dose in animals. However, again there was reluctance to exceed the equivalent NOAEL dose in man.

In two of the above examples, the top dose reached in the patient population was close to the NOAEL dose in animals. However, depending on the specific toxicologic findings in animals, there may be great reluctance to exceed the equivalent NOAEL dose in man, even when it appears that dose could be well tolerated in man. In such circumstances, we believe that the FDA or other agency should be consulted and, if agreed, higher doses should be tested in man in order to fully characterize the optimal dose range for efficacy trials. Next we will examine animal models from a pharmacokinetic standpoint.

ANIMAL MODELS FOR PHARMACOKINETICS

Although it is generally not possible to extrapolate all the pharmaco-kinetic parameters in humans from animal studies, reasonably good predictions can be made under certain conditions. In contrast to drug efficacy and toxicity, which depend on pharmacokinetic as well as pharmacodynamic factors such as receptor density and affinity, several pharmacokinetic parameters are more closely related to basic physiological processes. In cases where these physiological processes are similar across species and where there is an absence of confounding factors, animal models can be extrapolated to humans.

Physiological and Allometric Models

Two main approaches have been used to model pharmacokinetics across species. *Physiologically-based pharmacokinetic (PBPK) models* are mechanistic, attempting to model important anatomical, biochemical, and physiological features of each of the main tissues, thereby constructing a valid model of the entire organism. *Allometric models* are more empirical, examining relationships between size, time, and parameters of interest without necessarily considering the underlying mechanisms behind these relationships. Allometric models tend to be less detailed than physiological models.

Physiological models need to include structures/tissues that account for route of administration, major storage sites in the body (e.g. muscle, adipose tissues), tissues involved with elimination, and target tissues (Gabrielsson, 1991). The parameters *for each tissue* would include tissue size (volume/mass), tissue perfusion (blood/CSF flow rates), tissue partioning (equilibrium of drug between tissue and blood/CSF), protein binding, permeability/diffusion, drug metabolism, drug excretion, and in some cases drug formation (Ings, 1990; Gabrielsson 1991). By the time that 6 to 12 tissues are included in a model, it may become quite complex. Many of the values used in physiological models come from the literature or from *in vitro* experiments. As development continues, the results of successive experiments can be incorporated as feedback to refine the model. At its best, a physiological model can predict the varying concentrations of a drug in several different tissues over time with a detail that compartmental models could never match. If the model works, it is possible to calculate tissue exposures. However physiological models frequently don't work because there are too many variables. In addition, they are very time-consuming and difficult to construct. The main utility of physiological models lies in the examination of target organ exposures; often a model that is seriously lacking in some respects may still provide a good explanation for one component (Ings, 1990).

A relatively simple yet effective physiological model specific to the central compartment has been devised by Gabelnick and coworkers (1970) to describe the distribution of chloride between blood and brain. It includes 3 compartments: the brain (i.e. central compartment), a well-perfused compartment, and a poorly-perfused compartment. Blood flow rates between the well-perfused and the poorly perfused compartments are included, along with CSF flow between the well-perfused compartment and the brain. Mediated transport from the well-perfused compartment to the brain is included, along with diffusive transport between the two compartments. Finally, elimination from the well-perfused compartment is also considered. Obviously modeling of the distribution of an ion is an easier task than describing the fate of a drug that is metabolized, but Gabelnick's model illustrates that the complexity of a model should match its purpose.

Allometric scaling of data is more commonly practiced in drug development due to its relative simplicity. At the most empirical extreme there are "rules of thumb" such as "to predict toxicity scale a human dose as 1/12 the mouse dose (in mg/kg) and 1/7 the rat dose." Despite their empirical nature, allometric models can have considerable validity if they are based on physiological or anatomical principles. It is generally a good idea to test a drug in several species if an allometric equation will be used, especially in the more empirical situations, as one or two species can deviate considerably from the proposed relationship. In a comparison of 12 benzodiazepines in dogs and humans, for example, the rate of metabolic clearance varied between compounds from 3-fold faster in dogs to 72-fold faster in dogs (Boxenbaum, 1982). In fairness, it should be noted that drug metabolism and protein binding vary considerably from species to species and thus metabolic clearance is not a particularly good example of the utility of allometric scaling.

Allometric scaling is based on an equation of the form:

$$Y = aW^b$$

where Y is the variable being modeled, W is body weight, a is the allometric coefficient, and b is the allometric exponent. The allometric exponent is usually less than one; for example, liver weight has an allometric exponent of 0.85. This is because the relative size of the liver (and most other anatomical and physiological variables) decreases as the size of the animal increases. Although body weight is the most common variable for normalizing data, surface area (see previous discussion), liver weight, kidney weight, amount of enzyme, or other factors can be used as well (Lin 1995). As allometric relationships exist between these potential bases for normalization, conversion between systems is straightforward.

In practice, both allometric and physiological methods of modeling pharmacokinetics have drawbacks. As Lin (1995) states:

> Although both physiological and allometric methods are of academic interest, they are not practical and have only limited use in drug discovery and development. The former approach tends to be costly and time-consuming, with frequent failures in obtaining all the parameters needed. The latter is also costly and time-consuming, because it requires the kinetic data from at least four or five species to define the allometric relationship properly. Often, these kinetic parameters are not available before the initial clinical studies, which is the time when an accurate prediction of human pharmacokinetics is most needed. In fact, most of the reported literature successfully showing the animal-human prediction, particularly those based on an allometric approach, are essentially hindsight and not predictive.

The reader is referred to Lin's excellent review for a description of the utility of animal pharmacokinetic models from the viewpoint from the pharmaceutical industry. He describes a realistic approach, generally along the lines of allometric models, but with attention to mechanistic issues and the assessment of factors that may complicate interspecies extrapolation.

Calculation of Pharmacokinetic Parameters

A simplified list of the primary factors that influence pharmacokinetic parameters, based on Lin (1995), is shown in Table 2.2. It is important to emphasize that there are a number of other factors that can alter these variables. For example, absorption is a complex process that is influenced by the molecular size, shape, pKa, lipophilicity, solubility, and reactivity of the compound, as well as the dosing regimen and vehicle, the gastric and intestinal transit times, and fasting or fed state of the animal. Physiological factors such as the absorptive surface area, the cell types present, the regional flow of blood, and the pH also play a role (van Vliet, 1996; Lin, 1995). Fortunately the intrinsic absorption of compounds across the wall of the gastrointestinal tract is similar across species, so absorption can often be extrapolated if proper attention is paid to potential confounding factors. Thus it is important to investigate such things as pH differences in solubility in order to properly evaluate animal absorption data.

In preclinical bioavailability studies, perhaps the most critical assessment is the relative contribution of absorption and first-pass metabolism. First-pass metabolism is often species-specific and even varies from individual to individual, depending on genetics and diet. Metabolism also has the potential to be induced or saturated. In summary, Benet (1993) states "at this stage in our understanding of the various metabolic isozymes, it is necessary to actually carry out studies in man to ascertain that what is observed in the animal models is relevant to man".

In general, human pharmacokinetic parameters are most readily calculated from animal data when there is minimal first-pass metabolism, little protein binding, and high renal clearance. Physiological processes such as absorption of a compound across the wall of the gastrointestinal

Table 2.2 Factors that Influence the prediction of human pharmacokinetic parameters from animal data.

Parameter	Primary Factors	Predictability
Bioavailabilty (F)	Absorption	Good
	First-pass Metabolism	Poor
Clearance (Cl)		
Hepatic (low clearance)	Plasma Protein Binding	Poor
	Metabolism	Poor
Hepatic (high clearance)	Hepatic Blood Flow	Good
Renal	Glomerular Filtration Rate (GFR)	Good
Volume of	Volume of Body Water	Excellent
Distribution (V_d)	Plasma Protein Binding	Poor
	Tissue Protein Binding	Poor
Area Under the Curve (AUC)	F and Cl (See above)	Generally Poor
Half Life ($t_{1/2}$)	Cl and V_d (See above)	Generally Poor

tract (as discussed above) and glomerular filtration are relatively similar across species. An allometric equation or species-by-species scaling factors can be used for calculations. Protein binding and enzymatic metabolism, on the other hand, depend critically on protein amino acid sequences; a change of a single amino acid can dramatically alter the protein-drug interaction. Thus there is no a priori way to predict differences between species. *In vitro* studies of plasma and tissue protein binding are an important component in predicting drug distribution in humans, while *in vitro* metabolic studies are needed to assess the relevance of data generated from animal models. In addition, both protein binding and enzyme metabolism can also play a role in drug-drug interactions.

In considering CNS compounds, the fact that the peripheral and central compartments may not respond identically comes into play. It is important to remember that the pharmacokinetic profiles may differ between the blood and CSF. An understanding of the systemic pharmacokinetic profile is still invaluable in tracing mass-balance relationships, metabolism, and elimination. In addition, many adverse effects are peripheral in nature. Nevertheless, investigators should make efforts to understand the behavior of CNS compounds in the central compartment. Efforts to assess central response in humans in early clinical trials will be discussed in Chapter 5.

Regulatory and Design Issues

The importance of animal pharmacokinetic studies in the development of new drugs is generally not reflected in regulations, although it appears as though this will be addressed in the International Harmonization Guidelines. In the United States, for example, there are no specific federal regulations other than the requirement to include a section in the IND reporting the pharmacological effects, mechanisms of action, and ADME in animals, "if known" (Fitzgerald, 1993). Guidelines are not much more detailed, indicating that available data should be organized by species in the following order: absorption, pharmacokinetics, serum half-life, protein binding, tissue distribution/accumulation, enzyme induction or inhibition, and excretion pattern, and that doses should be clearly specified. As Glenna Fitzgerald (1993) states, "One might therefore have the impression that nonclinical pharmacokinetic and drug metabolism studies constitute a minor part of the overall characterization of a new drug. ... nothing could be further from the truth." It is clear that biokinetics are an essential part of the drug application process despite minimal regulatory restrictions. This is appropriate, as the utility of animal models varies from indication to indication and from compound to compound.

A conference report (Peck et al., 1992) offers a good consensus statement as to the type of information that "will often be of value", although it is important to emphasize that this report must not be construed as an official governmental position. The majority of the recommended preclinical studies, summarized in Table 2.3, are concerned with the measurement of pharmacokinetic variables, while the studies that focus on efficacy and toxicity pointedly relate these measures to drug concentration rather than dose.

Benet (1993) lists the 10 most important pharmacokinetic parameters to determine (in order of importance): clearance, effective concentration range, extent of availability, fraction of the available dose excreted unchanged, blood/plasma concentration ratio, half-life, toxic concentrations, extent of protein binding, volume of distribution, and rate of availability.

Table 2.3 Informative preclinical studies (Peck et al., 1992).

Develop methodologies for quantification of drug and metabolite concentrations in biologic
    fluids
Mass balance-metabolism profile and metabolic pharmacology
Pharmacokinetics and biological fluid concentration monitoring
Relation of systemic drug concentrations to pharmacodynamic endpoints
Systemic drug concentration monitoring in long-term toxicology studies
Protein binding
Tissue distribution
Placental transfer kinetic studies

DO ANIMAL MODELS FOR CNS CONDITIONS SERVE AS GOOD PREDICTORS OF CLINICAL EFFICACY?

An extensive number of animal models for CNS indications have been devised for the screening of new therapeutic agents and for the study of neuropsychiatric disorders. While animal models provide a valuable resource in the process of drug development, it is important to note that a number of therapeutic compounds including chlorpromazine and monoamine oxidase inhibitors have been developed without the benefit of animal models. The purpose of animal models therefore, is primarily to provide some understanding of the mechanism of action of new compounds and to provide a rationale for their use in a particular indication.

An ideal animal model is one in which the etiology, neuropathology, and symptomatology of the disease are reproduced. However, in the absence of a complete understanding of the neurobiological basis of many CNS disorders, most animal models of neuropsychiatric conditions have attempted to simulate various aspects of a given disease or disorder. Further, it is important to note that disorders involving behavioral and thought dysfunctions, such as schizophrenia, anxiety, and depression, are particularly difficult to model in an animal system.

Validity

Since animal behavior in the context of an animal model can be difficult to extrapolate to a human behavioral disorder, the validity of animal models for human disease must be assessed in order to ascertain whether a model is relevant to the clinical condition. The utility of a model in generating insight into the treatment of a disorder is inextricably linked to the validity of the model in reproducing the clinical condition. For example, a model which reproduces only one aspect of a complex disorder will repeatedly identify compounds with a similar mechanism of action; whereas a model which bears greater etiologic similarity to the condition is more likely to aid in the identification of a variety of novel therapeutic agents. Animal model validation is an ongoing process which evolves both with discovery of new compounds and with enhanced understanding of the condition being modeled.

An approach for evaluating the validity of an animal model based on analysis of its predictive, face, and construct validity has been described (Willner, 1995). A model with a high degree of predictive validity indicates that the model is responsive to established manipulations known to alter the pathology of the clinical disorder. Thus, drugs which are known to alleviate the symptoms of the disorder should have a similar effect in the model as in the patient. For certain classes of drugs, however, interspecies differences in metabolism, pharmacodynamics and pharmacokinetics can contribute to a lack of predictive validity.

Face validity refers to phenomenological similarities between the disorder and the model. A model with a high degree of face validity will demonstrate strong similarities in specific symptomatology, or at least will address a major symptom of the disorder. Because animals respond to stimuli with different behavioral output than animals, and because animals cannot report thoughts and feelings, it is important to design models which draw on commonalities between the species.

Construct validity is a measure of the theoretical rationale of the model. Construct validity is a assessment of how similar the behavior being modeled is to the actual behavior in the clinical condition in terms of its etiology and underlying cognitive origin. Due to the incomplete understanding of the theoretical foundation of many neuropsychiatric disorders, construct validity is difficult to demonstrate, but is considered a fundamental aspect of a sound animal model.

The determination of the validity of an animal model using the criteria of predictive, construct and face validity serves as a guide and useful exercise in evaluating the overall suitability of a model as a simulation of a human disorder. As advance are made in the understanding of these complex clinical conditions, more valid animal models may be devised. For example, early animal models of Alzheimer's disease focused on the deficiency in cholinergic transmission, the major symptom of the disease. These models were used to identify a class of therapeutic agents with activity on the cholinergic system. While these agents offered the first breakthrough in the treatment of Alzheimer's disease, cholinesterase inhibitors provide only a palliative therapy and do not affect the disease progression. However, the recent increased understanding of the role of possible genetic loci in the development of the disease has permitted the generation of transgenic models in which the pathogenic cascade may be more faithfully reproduced. Since these models may permit an accurate recreation of the disease, the potential for the identification of novel therapies in which the underlying cause of the disease may be interrupted will be greatly enhanced.

ANIMAL MODELS FOR ANXIETY

Based on the physiologic targets of anxiolytic compounds, numerous neurotransmitters and neuromodulators have been implicated in anxiety, including the GABA/benzodiazepine chloride ionophore complex, 5-HT_{1A}, 5-HT_2, and 5-HT_3, NMDA, cholecystokinin and others (Kulkarni and Reddy, 1996). More than 30 behavioral animal models for anxiety based on induced fear have been developed and used for the screening of compounds with anxiolytic activity. However, since the major criterion of a good animal model has been its sensitivity to known compounds (most notably the benzodiazepines), and not its ability to mimic the neurochemical basis of the clinical disorder, established models tend to identify compounds of like mechanism of action, rather than revealing distinct and novel agents.

Punishment/conflict

Punishment, or conflict models of anxiety have been widely used for the screening of compounds with potential anxiolytic activity. Numerous variations of this model have been described including the Vogel punished drinking test (Vogel et al, 1971), and punished operant responding (Geller and Seifter, 1960). Punishment or conflict models involve the administration of an aversive stimulus in response to a particular behavior. The conflict between the positive motivation to emit the behavior (typically hunger, thirst, or exploration) and the negative motivation (fear) of the punishment which will follow creates a situation thought to be analogous to clinical anxiety in the test animal. In an untreated animal, the frequency of response behavior is reduced following introduction of the aversive stimulus. The administration of anxiolytic compounds in the punishment model attenuates the avoidance behavior, increasing the frequency of response.

In the Vogel punished drinking model which has been frequently used in many preclinical tests of anxiolytic compounds, benzodiazepines were found to increase punished drinking. The limitations of this model are apparent when viewed in the context of the failure of a novel set of anxiolytic compounds, the azapirones, to elicit an alteration in the behavioral response of rats and monkeys to punished drinking. This class of compounds acts on $5\text{-}HT_{1A}$ receptors to reduce serotonergic transmission, in contrast to the benzodiazepines, which act on a component of the GABA receptor complex. Interestingly, the azapirones did produce an effect in a pigeon punished feeding model, indicating that species differences can affect outcome. These data emphasize the need to test new compounds in more than one species and in more than one model during preclinical testing.

Passive avoidance

Passive avoidance models have been frequently used to evaluate the potential clinical efficacy of anxiolytic compounds. In this model, when an animal attempts exploration of a chamber by stepping into an adjoining compartment, a shock is delivered. When the animal is retested, the subject avoids the exploratory response. The administration of buspirone prior to the retest causes an attenuation of the avoidance behavior in a dose-dependent manner (Sanger and Joly, 1990). In contrast, the benzodiazepines are unable to alter the avoidance behavior when administered after the initial learning phase (Sanger and Joly, 1985). Thus, the passive avoidance model is sensitive to compounds acting on the 5-HT receptors, but not the GABA receptor complex.

Potentiated startle response

Animal models for anxiety are thus intrinsically limited in their capacity to identify compounds of novel pharmacologic action because they are based on simple behavioral observations which fail to fully reproduce the neurochemical complexities inherent in a true clinical condition. In particular, some authors have noted the poor face validity of punishment models in so far as the behavior of animals trained in punishment procedures does not appear emotional, but rather, is appropriate and adaptive (Morgan, 1968, Millenson and Leslie, 1974).

The potentiated startle response (Brown et al., 1951) is a model which is considered by some investigators to more accurately reflect the emotion of anxiety. In this model, the subjects are presented with a neutral stimulus such as light, paired with an aversive stimulus such as shock. After the conditioning, the animals are then presented with a loud tone upon which the startle response is measured. When the tones are preceded by the conditioned stimulus, the startle response is potentiated. Significantly, many classes of anxiolytics, including the benzodiazepines (Davis,1979), buspirone and other 5-HT_{1A} agonists (Mansbach and Geyer, 1988), and ondansetron (a 5-HT_3 antagonist) (Glenn and Green, 1989) have been shown to block the potentiated startle response. While most compounds yielding anxiolytic activity in the model showed corresponding therapeutic value in human, ondansetron has not proven clinically useful in the treatment of anxiety (Bell and Deveaugh-Geiss, 1994). Thus, although the potentiated startle model has demonstrated improved predictive validity over conflict procedures with both classic and novel compounds, performance in the model does not correlate with all classes of anxiolytic compounds.

Social interaction test

Because it does not involve conditioning, deprivation or punishment, the social interaction test (File and Hyde, 1979) is considered a model which may more closely mirror human anxiety in the context of social phobias. In the social interaction test, unfamiliar pairs of rats are placed in various conditions and the extent of their social interaction measured. In anxiety-producing conditions, such as an unfamiliar chamber in bright light, social interaction is reduced. This response can be attenuated by the administration of anxiolytic compounds including the benzodiazepines as well as novel anxiolytics.

Elevated plus-maze

The elevated plus maze (Pelow, 1986) is a widely accepted and applied paradigm for the study of anxiety related behavior in rodents. The model is considered more relevant to situations which induce human anxiety, because it does not involve conditioned behavior or punishment procedures. When untreated rodents are placed in the center of an elevated plus sign-shaped maze with an open arm, they avoid movement into the open arm, presumably due to fear of height and open spaces.

Compounds including the benzodiazepines, buspirone, and ondansetron, have been demonstrated to decrease avoidance of the open arm, but results have been variable depending on the laboratory in which the experiments were performed, with roughly equal numbers of both positive and negative findings (reviewed in Rodgers 1997). Similarly, in the light-dark aversion test, anxiolytic compounds have been shown to reduce the avoidance of light. A novel anxiolytic, SC 48,274, which acts on receptors distinct from $5\text{-}HT_{1A}$ and GABA receptors, was found to be active in the elevated plus maze, the light-dark aversion test and in the social interaction test (Crawley, 1985; Cutler et al., 1996); however, clinical results were not promising (Cutler et al., 1994)

Although classic models such as conflict procedures are limited in their ability to identify novel anxiolytic compounds, models such as the social interaction test, the elevated plus maze, the light-dark aversion test, and the mirrored chamber test (Kulkarni and Reddy, 1996) have proved valuable in offering a testing ground for compounds acting on diverse receptors. Since the identification of multiple forms of anxiety disorder, the trend in creating new animals models has begun to lean toward addressing the individual subclasses, such as panic disorder, phobias, social interaction anxiety, and others. With increased understanding of the neurologic and genetic basis of anxiety, animal models which more faithfully reproduce the clinical condition will provide enhanced utility as a testing vehicle for novel agents.

ANIMAL MODELS FOR DEPRESSION

Major depressive disorder is differentiated from depression induced by a stressful event in its neurochemical basis (reviewed in Richardson, 1991). In the patient with major depressive disorder, depression results from an imbalance of neurochemical substrates responsible for mood. Neurotransmitters including dopamine, serotonin, acetylcholine and others have been implicated in major depressive disorder. In contrast, the patient who is depressed from a loss or stress, homeostatic mechanisms are intact. The distinction between these states is important for the design of appropriate animal models in which to investigate the action of novel drugs (Richardson, 1991). Since depression is a disorder characterized by behavioral and mood abnormalities which respond to medication, an animal model of depression should in turn exhibit disturbances similar to the patient which respond to antidepressant drugs.

Chronic mild stress-induced anhedonia

Anhedonia, or the inability to experience pleasure, is one of the core symptoms of depression. Animal models of anhedonia induced by chronic unpredictable mild stressors have been used to address this aspect of depression, and have been the most widely used and best validated animal models in the identification of compounds with antidepressant activity. In these models, the degree of anhedonia is measured by the rate of response to rewarding stimuli following a period of exposure to transient, intermittent stressful conditions, such as confinement, food or water deprivation, overcrowded housing, ringing bells, and reversed light/dark schedules.

The construct and face validity of the model are adequate, given the similarity of the behavioral condition (anhedonia) and the manner in which it is induced (chronic mild stress), to human clinical depression (Moreau et al., 1996). In addition, the predictive validity of the model has been established with tricyclic antidepressants, atypical antidepressants, reversible monoamine oxidase inhibitors, whereas non antidepressant drugs did not exert behavioral changes in the model (reviewed in Moreau et al., 1996). Recent reports also demonstrated the effects of two selective 5-HT$_{2C}$ receptor agonists in the anhedonia model (Moreau et al., 1996), and in rat and monkey models of obsessive-compulsive disorder (OCD) (Martin et al., 1995), suggesting the potential for therapeutic application of these compounds in clinical depression and OCD.

Learned helplessness

Learned helplessness models of depression may also be thought of as models of anxiety because the induction of the helpless response is dependant on the induction of anxiety, and anxiolytic compounds attenuate the conditioned behavior, as well as antidepressant compounds (Mineka and Zinbarg, 1996). The fundamental aspect of this model is very similar to stress-induced anhedonia in that inactivity results following conditioning with uncontrollable aversive stimuli.

Studies of the neurochemistry of the learned helplessness response have demonstrated a release of dopamine in response to stress, leading to increased release of serotonin. After the initial training phase in the learned helplessness model, animals have greater serotonin depletion; agents which act to increase serotonin levels thus attenuate the LH response. These data further support the validity of the LH model, since these same neurochemical changes and receptor alterations have been implicated in the clinical disorder (Anisman et al., 1991). It is important to note that response to antidepressants in the learned helplessness and anhedonia models is variable across different mouse strains, just as human interindividual response to treatment also varies (Shanks and Anisman, 1989).

Behavioral Despair

A widely used version of the behavioral despair model is the forced swimming test. In this model, the test animal is first placed in an inescapable cylinder of water for a period of 15 minutes. When animals are retested 24 hours later, the frequency of escape attempts is reduced; however, administration of antidepressants attenuates this "despair", and increases motility. The forced swimming test is sensitive to all the major classes of antidepressant drugs including the tricyclics, monoamine oxidase inhibitors, and atypical antidepressants (Detke et al., 1997), as well as some anxiolytic compounds such as buspirone.

Social separation/isolation

The social separation model of depression has been used predominantly in non-human primates as a loss-induced model of clinical depression. This model is analogous to the stress-induced anhedonia and learned helplessness model in that behavior following a period of social separation such as removing an infant from the mother, or social isolation in which the subject is isolated from its peers, resembles some aspects of clinical depression.

Olfactory bulbectomized rat

The olfactory bulbectomized (OBX) rat has been used as a model of depression (reviewed in Richardson, 1991). Removal of the olfactory bulb, which synthesizes a wide variety of neurotransmitters, creates a neurochemical imbalance, causing a constellation of symptoms analogous to major clinical depression. In tests of passive avoidance, OBX rats fail to modify their behavior in reaction to environmental stimuli. After chronic treatment with antidepressant compounds such as the classic tricyclic antidepressants, the selective serotonin reuptake inhibitors, and numerous novel antidepressants, OBX rats respond in a manner similar to non-bulbectomized animals. The predictive validity of the model is excellent, with the correct identification of over 18 compounds with antidepressant activity. Only 2 predictive errors have been made by the OBX rat model: one false positive and one false negative. In addition the construct and face validity of the model are very high, with many similarities in behavioral abnormalities, as well as similar disruptions in noradrenaline, serotonin, GABA, acetylcholine, and other neurotransmitters.

Flinders sensitive rats

The Flinders Sensitive Line (FSL) of rats is a genetic model for depression based on a cholinergic hyperfunction theory of depression (Overstreet et al., 1979). The administration of cholinergic agonists causes an exaggeration of existing symptoms in depressed patients (Overstreet et al., 1988). Therefore, investigators have postulated a role of the cholinergic system in depression, with cholinergic supersensitivity as a possible marker for depression. Like depressed patients, FSL rats exhibit decreases in limbic function including low body weight, reduced activity, and sleep abnormalities, and increased immobility upon exposure to stress (reviewed in Overstreet and Janowsky, 1991). The response to antidepressant drugs is less well characterized in the FSL rat than in the OBX rat; however, FSL rats do respond to imipramine and lithium. Because depression likely results from an interplay of several neurochemicals, one of which is acetylcholine, and because the disorder is heterogeneous in nature, the model may only address one aspect of a complicated neurological dysfunction.

ANIMAL MODELS FOR SCHIZOPHRENIA

Schizophrenia is difficult to model in animals due to its distinctly human attributes of delusion, hallucination, and thought disorder. Therefore, as with other behavioral abnormalities, animal models of schizophrenia have focused on specific individual aspects of the disorder.

Pharmacologically-induced psychosis

Amphetamine

The predominant hypothesis of the pathogenesis of schizophrenia is a defect in dopaminergic transmission, although recent investigation has pointed to potential differences in many neurotransmitter systems. The dopaminergic hypothesis was derived in part following observations of schizophrenic symptoms during administration of amphetamine which increases dopaminergic transmission in the CNS (Randrup and Munkvad, 1965). The amphetamine model provided a major contribution to the identification of typical neuroleptics including the phenothiazines and butyrphenones as treatments for schizophrenia. The most significant disadvantage of the neuroleptics in clinical practice has been the extrapyramidal symptoms (EPS) caused by blockade of D_2 receptors in motor neurons.

The predictive validity of the amphetamine model is poor for the atypical antipsychotic, clozapine (a $5\text{-}HT_2$ receptor antagonist), which is weak in its ability to antagonize amphetamine-induced stereotypic behavior (Bruhwyler et al., 1993). The major limitation of the amphetamine model is that the level of response is dependant on the affinity of the test compound for the D_2 dopamine receptors, such that compounds like clozapine, which bears only weak affinity for the D_2 receptors, respond poorly in the model. However, 5-HT receptor antagonists including fananserin, which binds both the $5\text{-}HT_{2A}$ receptor and D4 receptors with high affinity show activity in marmoset model of amphetamine-induced cognitive disturbance (Domeney et al., 1994). Activity in the amphetamine model is still used quite commonly in the assessment of new compounds with potential antipsychotic activity.

The development of the dopamine overactivation hypothesis of schizophrenia, and the success of the amphetamine model in identifying clinically useful compounds resulted in a profusion of animal models based on dopamine. Research in the last decade, however, has implicated the role of numerous other neurotransmitter systems in schizophrenia including serotonin, γ-aminobutyric acid (GABA), glutamate (and the NMDA receptor), aspartate, and acetylcholine. The goal of animal models in the future will be to more closely simulate the clinical condition by addressing as many aspects of the disorder as possible in a single model system. Recent work with the phencyclidine model of psychosis may prove to be a step in this direction.

Phencyclidine

Phencyclidine, or PCP, which was used as an early anesthetic and later as a street drug, was found to induce a set of thought disturbances in attention, perception, and symbolic thinking indistinguishable from schizophrenia, and not induced by amphetamines (Cohen et al., 1961). In particular, PCP produces a flat affect (one of the hallmark symptoms of schizophrenia), auditory hallucinations, the inability to maintain cognitive set, thought blocking, concreteness, and peculiar verbalizations (reviewed in Steinpresis, 1996) To date, the phencyclidine model of psychosis has received wide usage in the attempt to both gain insight into the neurobiological basis of schizophrenia and to identify novel therapeutic agents (Javitt and Zukin, 1991; Ogawa et al., 1994; Steinpresis, 1996). Studies with PCP have identified a site within the NMDA receptor complex as the target for the drug (Javitt and Zukin, 1991). Antipsychotic compounds including clozapine and haloperidol (Freed et al., 1980) yield varying degrees of activity against aspects of phencyclidine-induced psychosis. The phencyclidine model of psychosis will likely be of great utility in the identification of novel therapeutics for the neuroleptic resistant behavioral symptoms.

Behavioral models for psychosis

Latent Inhibition

Latent inhibition (LI) refers to the retarded conditioning that results after a stimulus has been previously presented without reinforcement. The LI response has been observed in many mammalian species, and is considered to operate in an analogous manner across species (Lubow and Gewirtz, 1995). LI is disrupted in acute schizophrenia and in amphetamine-treated rats and humans (Gray et al., 1992, Kilcross and Robbins, 1993), and enhanced only with drugs with known antipsychotic efficacy (Dunn et al., 1993), including the atypical antipsychotics clozapine (Weiner et al., 1996) and MDL 100,907. Therefore, the predictive, face, and validity of the model have been established (Weiner et al., 1996). As one of the major setbacks in the identification of novel compounds for the treatment of schizophrenia has been the failure of amphetamine animal models to respond to both neuroleptics and to atypical antipsychotics, the LI model offers improved predictive validity for a range of antipsychotic compounds and may prove useful in the evaluation of novel antipsychotic compounds.

Conditioned Avoidance

Disruption of conditioned avoidance behavior in nonhuman primates has been used as a predictor of the potential antipsychotic activity of new compounds (Heffner et al., 1989). Long lasting inhibition of conditioned avoidance in monkeys has been demonstrated with many antipsychotic compounds.

Hippocampal lesion models

The brains of schizophrenic patients are thought to bear abnormalities in hippocampal structure acquired during fetal development (reviewed in Schumajuk and Tyberg, 1991). Based on this theory, a number of animal models have been developed in which many aspects of schizophrenia are mimicked by the generation of surgically or chemically induced hippocampal brain lesions. A rat model of schizophrenia in which symptoms resembling schizophrenia emerge following adolescence has been developed by the introduction of ventral hippocampal neurotoxic lesions in the neonate (Lipska et al., 1993). In this model, ibotenic acid-lesioned rats exhibit a number of symptoms thought to be relevant to schizophrenia such as hypersensitivity to stress and amphetamine which improve upon treatment with haloperidol (Lipska et al., 1993). Ibotenic acid-lesioned rats also showed learning and memory deficits prior to puberty which may provide a early marker for prediction of the emergence of schizophrenia (Chambers et al., 1996). Others have proposed the use of kainic acid-lesioned rats as a potential model of schizophrenia (Bardgett et al., 1995). The validity of the lesion model is still in question and it remains to be seen whether this model will prove valuable in the study of schizophrenia and in the development of therapeutic agents for the disorder. As the nature of the abnormality in hippocampal structure in schizophrenic brains are better understood, it may be possible to create a lesion model which mirrors the neuropathogenesis of the disorder.

Motor activity

Various tests of motor activity including apomorphine-induced climbing, 5-hydroxytryptamine (5-HTP)-induced head twitching, and catalepsy induction are often used to establish the activity of a new compound against specific receptor types. Climbing behavior has been shown to require both D_1 and D_2 receptor activity; therefore inhibition of climbing indicates dopamine antagonist activity. The recently marketed antipsychotic olanzapine, which has dopamine antagonist activity (Bymaster et al., 1995), inhibited climbing behavior twice as effectively as clozapine. Typical antipsychotics such as haloperidol effectively inhibit climbing behavior at low concentrations. 5-HTP-induced head twitching is thought to be a measure of activity at the $5-HT_2$ receptors. Atypical antipsychotic compounds show high activity at low doses in this model relative to the neuroleptic drugs. The ability to induce catalepsy has also been used as a measure of D_2 receptor activity. Atypical antipsychotics, such as clozapine, olanzapine, and risperidone which have low affinity for the D_2 receptors do not cause catalepsy at doses required to inhibit behavioral responses in animal models (Baldwin and Montgomery, 1995). Neuroleptic compounds, on the other hand are well-know for their ability to induce catalepsy at low doses.

ALZHEIMER'S DISEASE

The predominant symptom of Alzheimer's disease (AD) is cognitive dysfunction due to a loss of cholinergic neurons in the basal forebrain. The only approved class of therapeutic compounds for AD are cholinesterase inhibitors which act to improve memory and learning by boosting cholinergic transmission. Agents such as these have been tested in animal behavioral models in which retention of learned behaviors, or learning of new information is measured. Both aged animals and scopolamine-lesioned animals have been subjected to behavioral examination in classic avoidance conditioning, maze tests, and reward paradigms.

Aged animals

Aged individuals of many species including rodents, rabbits, dogs, and monkeys have been used as animal models for Alzheimer's disease. While rodents demonstrate deficits in memory and learning similar to aged humans, the physical characteristics of neuritic plaques and neurofibrillary tangles are not found. Despite the failure of aged rodents to develop classic AD neuropathology, these animals do provide a model of cognitive dysfunction as measured by the ability of cholinergic agents to attenuate the learning and memory deficits observed in behavioral conditioning tests. Aged monkeys exhibit the greatest similarities in brain and behavioral abnormalities to humans (Martin et al., 1991; Rapp et al., 1989). However, due to the cost and difficulty in working with large animal models, the development of a rodent model continues to be a goal in the study of AD and in the development of novel therapeutics.

Lesion models

Preclinical studies of cholinesterase agents including cholinesterase inhibitors and muscarinic agonists have relied heavily on CNS-lesioned animal and human models of cholinergic dysfunction. Direct surgical lesions have not been widely used because the extent of the damage induced is beyond the bounds of the cholinergic system (Hanin, 1992). Excitatory amino acids, such as kainic or ibotenic acids, have been injected into CNS regions rich in cholinergic neurons (e.g. the basal nucleus of Meynert) with resultant cell death and degeneration of cholinergic projections to the area (Coyle, 1987). However, it is important to note that these chemical lesions cause widespread damage to dopamingeric neurons as well, and have been used as a model for schizophrenia as discussed above.

The most widely used lesion model for AD is the scopolamine-induced behavioral lesion which has the advantage of reversibility relative to surgical lesions, and has been employed in both animals and humans as a means of testing the ability of cholinomimetic compounds to reverse the lesion-induced cognitive deficits (Bartus, 1978; Flood and Cherkin, 1986; Dawson et al., 1991). Scopolamine, a muscarinic antagonist which causes temporary cognitive dysfunction, creates memory impairment in rats in passive and conditioned avoidance tests. The effects of the compound can be reversed by administration of relatively low doses of a wide variety of cholinesterase inhibitors and muscarinic agonists (Smith, 1988). In contrast, low doses of the agents are ineffective in the treatment of AD in humans, where only very high doses have been found to exert improvements in cognitive function. These findings emphasize the complexity of the disease process in AD, which involves defects in multiple neurotransmitters in addition to abnormalities of the amyloid and tau proteins, in contrast to the relatively simplistic nature of the scopolamine lesion, which is confined to a cholinergic deficit.

Transgenic models

While aged animals have been used as models for Alzheimer's disease, it is important to note that AD is more than simply an normal aging process of the brain. AD is a distinct neurodegenerative disease in which multiple genetic loci have been implicated. In the last decade, many attempts at producing mouse models of AD using transgenic technology have been reported. The relevance of these models to AD has been debated, as some models only partially reproduce the hallmark neuropathology and cognitive deficits. Differences in the selection of genes, alleles, and construct design as well as level of transgene expression and host strain all contribute to the vast differences observed in transgenic strains produced in different laboratories (Duff, 1997). Thus the determination of appropriate parameters necessary to induce AD in transgenic models is a difficult obstacle which will require extensive research. One recent β-amyloid transgenic model (Hsiao et al., 1996) in which a mutated β amyloid precursor protein was overexpressed, demonstrated both β-amyloid plaques and deficits in learning and memory with delayed onset. Models containing mutated presenilin transgenes (Duff et al., 1996; Citron et al., 1997) (also implicated in familial forms of AD) may also be useful in elucidating AD pathology. While transgenic models for AD are still being developed and characterized, this genre of animal model clearly represents the greatest hope in achieving better understanding of the AD disease process and in the development of novel therapeutic approaches.

ANIMAL MODELS FOR PARKINSON'S DISEASE

Parkinson's disease is a neurodegenerative motor function disorder in which nigral dopaminergic neurons are lost. The symptoms of the disease have been successfully treated with neurotransmitter replacement therapy; however, the degeneration continues during treatment and advanced stage patients suffer motor response fluctuations and dyskinesias. Evolving strategies for the treatment of PD include tissue transplantation and gene therapy. Successful embryonic allografting of DA neurons has been achieved in a small number of patients in early clinical trials (Freed et al., 1992; Kordower et al., 1995). However, graft rejection and controversy over the use of fetal tissue pose a complication in the treatment of PD with neural allografts (Borlongan et al., 1996). Although the gene responsible for the familial form of PD has not yet been cloned, gene therapy strategies using genes which facilitate dopaminergic transmission or which preserve dopaminergic neurons are under investigation (Mouradian and Chase, 1997).

Lesion models for PD are well-established and have shown excellent predictive, face, and construct validity. These include the 6-hydroxydopamine lesion of nigral neurons in rats, and the 1-methyl-4-phenyl-1,2,3-tetrahydropyridine (MTPT) lesion of nigral neurons in mice and non-human primates. In lesion models of hemiparkinsonism, destruction of dopaminergic neurons is created via the unilateral injection of chemical agents. The administration of dopamine agonists induces rotation away from the lesioned side, and has been used to predict the efficacy of new compounds. Non-human primate models have proven superior predictors of efficacy in humans than rat models. For example, while the partial D-1 agonist, SKF 38393 was effective in the rat PD model, it failed to attenuate experimental parkinsonism in the primate MPTP-lesion model (Bedard and Boucher, 1989; Falardeau et al., 1988). The D-1 agonist, CY 208-243 which demonstrated an effect in primates was subsequently found efficacious in PD patients (Emre et al., 1992;Temlett et al., 1989). While lesion induced animal models of PD have, in general, demonstrated excellent predictive validity for established antiparkinsonian agents, their validity in predicting the efficacy of transplantation and gene therapeutic strategies is still being determined. One criticism of the lesion induced models is that they fail to reproduce the slow degenerative nature of the neuronal loss in PD. Cloning of the PD gene will provide an advance in the ability to create more valid animal models via transgenic technology.

DO ANIMAL MODELS ACCURATELY PREDICT EFFECTIVE DOSES IN PATIENTS?

Preclinical studies of potential new compounds in animal models are beneficial in determining the potential efficacy of a possible treatment. The ability of an animal model to yield predictive data for the human depends on a number of factors. Most significantly, the similarity of the model to the human disease or disorder plays a substantial role in determining the correlation to humans. Compounds affecting the central nervous system are in general less predictive in animal models than systemic compounds (Spilker, 1991). Other factors include species differences in metabolism of the test compounds and in receptors for the compound, strain differences, and differences in toxicity which can potentially prevent the administration of therapeutic doses in humans. In addition, data obtained in animal models may differ depending on the laboratory in which it was generated, just as data obtained in human trials sometimes varies depending on the site at which they were performed. A large number of variables, such as population demographics, mode of administration, and differences in diagnostic criteria can contribute to variability of results in studies of human subjects.

Animal models of neuropsychiatric disease have been used with varying degrees of success to predict efficacy in human patients. Both false positives and false negatives can be demonstrated in many models and for particular compounds in certain types of models. Some examples of false positive and false negatives have been discussed in the preceding section. In some cases, a certain model is more heavily relied on than others for tests of efficacy in a particular indication. Because false positives are more desirable during the initial screening process, this model will not likely be the first tested (Spilker, 1991). It is also more likely that the compound will be first tested in lower animals such as rodents, prior to testing in higher species.

The process of extrapolating a effective dose from animal models to humans involves testing a compound under variety of conditions including route of administration, acute versus chronic exposure, timing of administration (for example in models of conditioned behavior, administration of the test compound can be conducted before or after initial conditioning, with varying effects on efficacy during the test phase), and single versus multiple dose panel testing. Multiple dose panel testing can be used to create a dose-response curve from which the dose which yields 50% response (ED_{50}) can be calculated. Blood levels of the test compound at the ED_{50} are often measured in order to provide prediction of plasma concentrations of effective doses in humans.

The selection of potentially therapeutic doses may be facilitated by the creation of a test battery in which effective doses in a particular animal model are correlated with the established effective dose range in patients. By establishing such a profile, the effective dose of a new compound with similar mechanism of action could be predicted in humans based on performance in the model.

Migraine

The animal saphenous vein model has been used with great accuracy to predict new anti-migraine compound efficacy and dosing in humans. In this model, preparations of saphenous veins are made from the species of choice, including the dog, rabbit, pig, or primate. Activity in this model is considered to be mediated by the $5\text{-}HT_{1D}$ receptor. Established anti-migraine compounds such as sumatriptan, a $5\text{-}HT_{1D}$ beta receptor agonist, induce measurable contraction in animal saphenous veins. The concentration of a new compound required to induce contraction in the model (as measured by the EC_{50}) can then be nearly directly translated into a concentration of the new compound in man. Thus in this manner, the saphenous vein model permits close approximation of an effective dose of a new compound in humans.

Anxiolytic Compounds

Benzodiazepines are effective in animal models of anxiety including punishment and conflict procedures, elevated mazes, social interaction tests. It is important to note, however, that since benzodiazepine sensitivity has long been the standard by which a new model for anxiety is measured, the majority of models respond to this class of anxiolytic compounds. The ED_{50} for 3 benzodiazepine compounds in different animal models of anxiety along with the corresponding average daily doses used to treat patients with

Table 2.3   Effective doses of benzodiazepines in animal models of anxiety versus humans

Benzodiazepine	ED_{50} in Rodent Model	Average Dose Range in Humans*
alprazolam	3 mg/kg (Sanger, 1991) punished eating	0.2 - 0.6 mg/kg
chlordiazepoxide	10 mg/kg (Sanger, 1990) punished operant responding	0.06 - 0.6 mg/kg
diazepam	1-2 mg/kg (Sanger 1991) staircase test	0.01 - 0.02 mg/kg

* Adapted from Cutler et al., 1996.

anxiety are listed in Table 2.3. These data show that effective doses of benzodiazepines are generally 10-fold lower in humans than those found effective in animal models of anxiety.

The novel anxiolytic compound, buspirone, is effective in animal models of anxiety and depression including the passive avoidance model, the potentiated startle response, the elevated plus-maze, and the forced swimming test. Effective doses (ED_{50}) in the animal models ranged from 2.5 to 5.0 mg/kg (reviewed in Sanger, 1991), while effective doses in humans are approximately 30 mg/day or about 0.44 mg/kg/day. Thus effective doses of buspirone in humans are about 5-10 fold lower than those in rodent models of anxiety.

Antipsychotics

In models of conditioned avoidance, ED_{50} values of typical and atypical antipsychotics have been determined for both rats and monkeys. Data obtained in a rat conditioned avoidance model (Moore et al., 1992) in which ED_{50} values were calculated for haloperidol, olanzapine, and clozapine, showed variability in prediction of effective doses in humans (Table 2.4). While effective doses in the rat model were 10-50+ fold higher than effective doses in humans for olanzapine and clozapine, effective doses of haloperidol in the rat model were similar to effective doses in humans.

In contrast to values obtained in the rat model, when ED_{50} values for a wide number of antipsychotic compounds were determined in monkey conditioned avoidance tests, values corresponded to effective doses in humans for most compounds tested within 2-3 fold. Thus the predictability of effective doses of antipsychotic compounds in conditioned avoidance models is superior in nonhuman primates compared to rodents.

Table 2.5 Comparison of Effective Doses of Antipsychotics: Rat vs Human

Antipsychotic	ED_{50} in rat conditioned avoidance*	Dose range in humans**
olanzapine	4.7 mg/kg	0.07 - 0.3 mg/kg/day
clozapine	21.3 mg/kg	0.4 - 1.5 mg/kg/day
haloperidol	0.5 mg/kg	0.03-0.6 mg/kg/day

*Moore et al., 1992
**Adapted from Sramek et al., 1996

The application of animal models in the prediction of effective doses in human is a difficult endeavor due to interspecies differences as well as varying degrees of suitability of the model as a means of reproducing the human neurological or psychiatric condition. The use of multiple models and species during preclinical screening aids in the identification of effective compounds. As emphasized in the examples shown above, nonhuman primate models tend to allow closer approximation of appropriate doses in humans.

In general, animal models do not reliably predict effective doses in humans, because conversion factors based on weight are simply inadequate. It is important to also note that in man, significant differences are found in tolerated doses between normal individual and patients, requiring the performance of bridging studies (see chapter 5). Thus the determination of effective doses in patients is the primary concern of Phase II trials. Appropriate Phase II study design is the only proven means of determining effective doses of new compounds. However, animal models can in some cases provide a guide for designing dose panels in clinical trials. By testing a panel of established compounds in a model and then comparing effective doses in the model with known effective doses in patients, a profile of response can be generated. When new compounds are tested in the model, comparison with known compounds can aid in dose extrapolation. On occasion, a compound which demonstrated activity in all established models in a given therapeutic area may not prove efficacious in humans. This can be explained by the failure to find an appropriate dose in humans, interspecies pharmacokinetic or pharmacodynamic differences, or failure of the models to adequately mimic the human disorder. As understanding of clinical conditions improves, it may be possible, as has been achieved in the testing of anti-migraine compounds, to design models which more accurately represent the desired disorder and hence provide more accurate dose prediction.

CONCLUSIONS: THE FUTURE OF ANIMAL MODELS FOR CNS INDICATIONS

In single gene disorders where inheritance follows in a Mendelian fashion, molecular genetic approaches may be used to identify the precise nature of the defect. When this information is obtained, animal models can be produced using transgenic technology. While the generation of an animal model using transgenic animals is a complicated task as illustrated by the struggle to create animal models for Alzheimer's disease, transgenic models can be powerful tools in both the dissection of the pathogenesis of the disease as well as in the identification of therapeutic compounds.

For neuropsychiatric disorders such as anxiety, depression, and schizophrenia which do not appear to be single gene defects based on inheritance patterns, the generation of animal models which reproduce the human disorder will continue to present a challenge. Despite the lack of Mendelian forms of psychiatric conditions, a genetic contribution to the etiology of these disorders has been implicated by family, twin and adoption studies (Risch, 1994; McGuffin, 1995). Recent studies have identified a possible role for a variant allele of the 5-HT_{2A} receptor in schizophrenia (Harrison and Geddes, 1996), and for an allele of the benzodiazepine receptor in the GABA-A complex in anxiety (Culiat et al., 1994). In view of the well-known participation of the GABA receptors in anxiety based on the response to benzodiazepines, genetic alterations in the GABA receptor complex may be linked to anxiety and other psychiatric disorders. Similarly, serotonin receptors play a role in anxiety, depression, and schizophrenia based on the response to compounds which regulate serotonergic transmission, suggesting a possible role for serotonin receptor allelic variants. Genetic polymorphisms may in addition permit identification of susceptibility factors or therapeutic subgroups (Mohler, 1997).

Animal models provide an invaluable resource for the study of neuropsychiatric disorders and for the identification of potential therapeutic agents. These models permit manipulation not possible in humans and protect the health and safety of human subjects. Many animal models have successfully identified agents with therapeutic value in humans. As animal models improve in their ability to mimic human conditions, the identification of novel therapies is enhanced and facilitated.

REFERENCES

21 CFR 1.312; 1992. Department of Health and Human Services, Food and Drug Administration Investigational New Drug Application, Revised as of April 1, 1992, Federal Register (special edition).

Alder S. Zbinden G. National and international drug safety guidelines. Zollikon, Switzerland: MTC Verlag, 1988.

Anisman H, Zalcman S, Shanks N, Zacharko RM. Multisystem regulation of performance deficits induced by stressors: an animal model of depression. In: Boulton A, Baker G, Martin-Iverson M, eds. *Neuromethods, Vol 19: Animal Models in Psychiatry.* Humana Press: Clifton, New Jersey, 1991: 1–59.

Auletta CS. Acute, Subchronic, and Chronic Toxicology. In: Derelanko MJ, Hollinger MA, eds. *CRC Handbook of Toxicology.*

Baldwin DS, Montgomery SA. First clinical experience with olanzapine (LY-170053): results of an open-label study and dose-ranging study in patients with schizophrenia. *Int Clin Psychopharmacol* 1995; **10**: 239–44.

Ball SE, Scatina JA, Sisenwine SF, Fisher GL. The application of in vitro models of drug metabolism and toxicity in drug discovery and drug development. *Drug Chemical Toxicology* 1995; **18**(1): 1–28.

Bardgett ME, Jackson JL, Taylor GT, Csernansky JG. Kainic acid decreases hippocampal neuronal number and increases dopamine receptor binding in the nucleus accumbens: an animal model of schizophrenia. *Behavioral Brain Research* 1995; **70**: 153-164.

Bartus R. Evidence for a direct cholinergic involvement in the scopolamine-induced amnesia in monkeys: effects of concurrent administration of physostigmine and methylphenidate with scopolamine. *Pharmacol Biochem Behav* 1978; **9**: 833–836.

Bedard PJ, Boucher R. Effect of D1 receptor stimulation in normal and MPTP monkeys. *Neurosci Lett* 1989; **104**: 223–228.

Bell J, Deveaugh-Geiss J. Multicenter trial of a 5-HT$_{3+}$ antagonist, ondansetron in social phobia. Presented at the *33rd Annual Meeting of the American College of Neuropsychopharmacology*; Dec 12-16, 1994; San Juan, Puerto Rico.

Benet LZ. The role of pharmacokinetics in the drug development process. In: Yacobi A, Skelly JP, Shah VP, Benet LZ, eds. *Integration of Pharmacokinetics, Pharmacodynamics, and Toxicokinetics.* New York: Plenum Press, 1993.

Borlongan CV, Stahl CE, Cameron DF, Saporta S, Freeman TB, Cahill DW, Sanberg PR. CNS immunological modulation of neural graft rejection and survival. *Neurol Res* 1996; **18**: 297–304.

Boxenbaum H. Comparative pharmacokinetics of benzodiazepines in dog and man. *J Pharmacokinet Biopharm* 1982; **10**: 411-426.

Brown JS, Kalish HI, Farber IE. Conditioned fear as revealed by magnitude of startle response to an auditory stimulus. *J Exp Psychol* 1951;**41**:317-328.

Bruce RD. A confirmatory study of the up-and-down method for acute toxicity testing. *Fundamental and Applied Toxicology* 1987; 8: 97-100.

Bruce RD. An up-and-down procedure for acute toxicity testing. *Fundamental and Applied Toxicology* 1985; 5: 151–157.

Bruhwyler J, Chkeide E, Houbeau G, Waegeneer N, Mercier M. Differentiation of haloperidol and clozapine using a coplex operant schedule in the dog. *Pharmacol Biochem Behav* 1993; 44: 181–189.

Bymaster FP, Hemrick-Lueke SK, Perry KW, Fuller RW. Neurochemical evidence for antagonism by olanzapine of dopamine, serotonin, alpha1-adrenergic and muscarinic receptors in vivo in rats. *Psychopharmacol* 1996; 124: 87–94.

Calabrese EJ. *Principles of Animal Extrapolation*. New York: Wiley, 1983.

Cereghino JJ, Kupferberg HJ. Preclinical Testing. In: French JA, Dichter MA, Leppik IE, eds., New Antiepileptic Drug Development: *Preclinical and Clinical Aspects. Epilepsy Res* 1993; Suppl 10: 19–30.

Chambers RA, Moore J, McEvoy JP, Levin ED. Cognitive effects of neonatal hippocampal lesions in a rat model of schizophrenia. *Neuropsychopharmacology* 1996; 15(6): 587–94.

Choudary J, Contrera JF, DeFelice A, DeGeorge JJ, Farrelly JG, Fitzgerald G, Goheer MA, Jacobs A, Jordan A, Meyers L, et al. Response to Monro and Mehta proposal for use of single-dose toxicology studies to support single-dose studies of new drugs in humans. *Clin Pharmacol Ther* 1996; 59: 265–7.

Citron M, Westaway D, Xia W, Carlson G, Diehl T, Levesque G, Johnson-Wood K, Lee M, Seubert P, Davis A, et al. Mutant presenilins of Alzheimer's disease increase production of 42-residue amyloid beta-protein in both transfected cells and transgenic mice. *Nat Med* 1997;3:67-72.

Cohen BD, Rosenbaum G, Luby ED, Gottlieb JS. Comparison of phencyclidine hydrochloride (Sernyl) with other drugs. *Arch Gen Psychiatry* 1961;6: 79–85.

Coyle JT. Excitotoxins. In: Meltzer H ed. *Psychopharmacology: The Third Generation of Progress,* Raven Press: New York, 1987: 333–340

Crawley JN. Exploratory behavior models of anxiety in mice. *Neurosci Biobehav Rev* 1985; 9: 37–44.

Crouch AEC. Tox_Risk: A program for fitting dose-response formulae and extrapolating between species. *Risk Analysis* 1989; 9(4): 599–603.

Cutler NR, Sramek JJ, Greenblatt DJ, Chaikin P, Ford F, Lesko LJ, Davis B, Williams RL. Defining the maximum tolerated dose: investigator, academic, industry and regulatory perspectives. *J Clin Pharmacol* 1997; 37: 767–783.

Cutler NR, Sramek JS, Kurtz NM. *Anxiolytic compounds: perspectives in drug development.* Wiley: Chichester, England, 1996.

Cutler NR, Sramek JS, Mac Pherson AE, An evaluation of the anxiolytic SC 48,274 in generalized anxiety disorder (GAD). *Prog Neuropsychopharmacol Biol Psychiatry* 1994; 18: 685–694.

Davis M. Diazepam and flurazepam: effects on conditioned fear as measured with the potentiated startle paradigm. *Psychopharmacol* 1979; 62: 1–7.

Dawson GR, Bentley G, Draper F, Rycroft W, Iverson SD, Pagella PG. The behavioral effects of heptylphysostigmine, a new cholinesterase inhibitor, in test of long-term and working memory in rodents. *Pharmacol Biochem Behav* 1991; **39**: 865–871

Detke MJ, Johnson J, ucki I. Acute and chronic antidepressant drug treatment in the rat forced swimming test model of depression. Exp *Clin Psychopharmacol* 1997; **5**: 107–112

Domeney AM, Mason SB, Costall B. Reversal learning impairments induced by amphetamine in the marmoset are attenuated by 5-HT receptor antagonists. *Brit J Pharmacol* 1994; **111**: 163.

Duff K, Alzheimer transgenic mouse models come of age. *Trends Neurosci* 1997; **20**: 279–280.

Duff K, Hardy J. Alzheimer's disease. Mouse model made. *Nature* 1995; **373**: 523–527.

Dunn LA, Atwater GE, Kilts CD. Effects of antipsychotic drugs on latent inhibition---sensitivity and specificity of animal behavioral model of clinical drug action. *Psychopharmacology* 1993; **112**: 315–323.

Emre M, Rinne UK, Rascol A, Lees A, Agid Y, LaTaste, X. Effects of a selective D1 agonist, CY 208-234, in de novo patients with Parkinson's disease. *Mov Disord* 1992; **7**: 239–243.

Falardeau P, Bouchard S, Bedard PJ, Boucher R, Di Paolo T. Behavioral and biochemical effect of chronic treatment with D-1 and D-2 dopamine agonists in MPTP-treated monkeys. *Eur J Pharmacol* 1988; **150**: 59–66.

File SE, Hyde JRG. A test of anxiety that distinguishes between the actions of benzodiazepines and those of other minor tranquilizers and of stimulants. *Pharmacol Biochem Behav* 1979; **11**: 65–68.

Fitzgerald GG. Pharmacokinetics and drug metabolism in animal studies (ADME, protein binding, mass balance, animal models). In: Yacobi A, Skelly JP, Shah VP, Benet LZ, eds. *Integration of Pharmacokinetics, Pharmacodynamics, and Toxicokinetics.* New York: Plenum Press, 1993.

Flood J, Cherkin A. Scopolamine effects on memory retention in mice: a model of dementia? *Behav Neural Biol* 1986;**45**:169-184.

Frazier JM. Update on validation. In: Goldberg AM, ed. *In Vitro Toxicology: Mechanisms and New Technology.* New York: Mary Ann Liebert, 1991, p. 179.

Freed CR, Breeze RE, Rosenberg NL, Schneck SA, Kriek E, Qi J-X, Lone T, Zhang Y-B, Snyder JA, Wells TH, et al. Survival of implanted dopamine cells and neurologic improvement 12 ot 46 months after transplantation for Parkinson's disease. *New Eng J Med* 1992; **327**: 1549–1555.

Freed WJ, Weinberger DR, Bing LA, Wyatt RJ. Neuropharmacological studies of phencyclidine (PCP)-induced behavioral stimulation in mice. *Psychopharmacology* 1980; **71**: 291–297.

Freireich EJ, Gehan E, Rall D, Schmidt L, Skipper L. Quantitative comparison of toxicity of anticancer agents in mouse, rat, hamster, dog, monkey and man. *Cancer Chemother Rep* 1966; **50**: 219–244.

Gabelnick HL, Dedrick RL, and Bourke RS. *In vivo* mass transfer of chloride during exchange hemodialysis. *J Appl Physiol* 1970; **28**: 636–640.

Gabrielsson JL. Utilization of physiologically based models in extrapolating pharmacokinetic data among species. *Fundam Appl Toxicol* 1991; **16**: 230–232.

Geller I, Seifter J. The effects of meprobamate, d-amphetamine and promazine on experimentally induced conflict in the rat. *Psychopharmacologia* 1960; **1**: 482–492.

Glenn B, Green S. Anxiolytic profile of GR 38032F in the potentiated startle paradigm. *Behav Pharmacol* 1989; **1**: 91–94.

Gonzalez FJ. Human cytochrome P450: problems and prospects. *Trends in Pharmacol Sci* 1992; **13**: 346.

Gray NS, Hemsley DR, Gray JA. Abolition of latent inhibition in acute, but not chronic schizophrenics. *Neurol Psychiat Brain Res* 1992; **1**:83–89.

Guengerich FP. Characterization of human cytochrome P450 enzymes. *FASEB J* 1992; **6**: 745.

Guidance for Industry: Single dose acute toxicity testing for pharmaceuticals. Center for Drug Evaluation and Research (CDER); August 1996.

Hanin I. Cholinergic toxins and Alzheimer's disease. *Ann NY Acad Sci* 1992; **11**: 63–70.

Heffner TG, Downs DA, Meltzer LT, Wiley JN, Williams AE. CI-943, a potential antipsychotic agent. I. Preclinical behavioral effects. *J Pharmacol Exp Ther* 1989; **251**: 105–112.

Heywood R. Prediction of adverse drug reactions from animal safety studies. In Bostrom H and Ljungstedt N, eds. *Detection and Prevention of Adverse Drug Reactions*. (Scandia International Symposia). Stockholm: Almqvist and Wiksell International, pp. 173–189.

Houston JB. Utility of in vitro drug metabolism data in predicting in vivo metabolic clearance. *Biochem Pharmacol* 1994; 47: 1469.

Hsiao K, Chapman P, Nilsen S, Eckman C, Harigaya Y, Younkin S, Yang F, Cole G. Correlative memory deficits, Aβ elevation, and amyloid plaques in transgenic mice. *Science* 1996; **274**: 99–102.

Ings RMJ. Interspecies scaling and comparisons in drug development and toxicokinetics. *Xenobiotica* 1990; **20**: 1201–1231.

International Conference on Harmonization of Technical Requirements for Registration of Pharmaceuticals for Human Use (ICH). Guidelines for Industry. Toxicokinetics: The assessment of systemic exposure in toxicity studies. Federal Register, March 1995.

Javitt DC, Zukin SR. Recent advances in the phencyclidine model of schizophrenia. *Am J Psychiatry* 1991; **148**: 1301–1308.

Johnsson G, Åblad B, Hansson E. Prediction of adverse drug reactions in clinical practice from animal experiments and phase I-II studies. In: Bostrom H and Ljungstedt N, eds. *Detection and Prevention of Adverse Drug Reactions.* (Scandia International Symposia). Stockholm: Almqvist and Wiksell International, pp. 190–99.

Killcross AS, Robbins TW. Differential effects of intra-accumbens and systemic amphetamine on latent inhibition using an on-baseline, within-subject conditioned suppression paradigm. *Psychopharmacology (Berl)* 1993; **110**(4): 479–489.

Kordower JH, Freeman TB, Snow B, Vingerhoets FJ, Muffson EJ, Sanberg PR, Hauser R, Perl DP, Olanow CW. Neuropathological evidence of graft survival and striatal reinnervation after transplantation of fetal mesencephalic tissue in a patient with Parkinson's disease. *New Eng J Med* 1995; **332**: 1118–1124.

Krasowskij GN. Extrapolation of experimental data from animals to man. *Environ Health Perspect* 1976; **13**: 51–58.

Kulkarni SK, Reddy DS. Animal behavioral models for testing antianxiety agents. *Meth Find Exp Clin Pharmacol* 1996; **18**: 219–230.

Lin J. Species similarities and differences in pharmacokinetics. *Drug Metab Dispos* 1995; **23**: 1008–1021.

Lipska BK, Jaskiw GE, Weinberger DR. Postpubertal emergence of hyperresponsiveness to stress and to amphetamine after neonatal excitotoxic hippocampal damage: a potential animal model of schizophrenia. *Neuropsychopharmacology* 1993; **9**: 67–75.

Litchfield JT Jr. Evaluation of the safety of new drugs by means of tests in animals. *Clin Pharmacol Ther* 1962; **3**: 665–672.

Lubow RE, Gerwitz JC. Latent inhibition in humans: Data, theory, and implications for schizophrenia. *Psychol Bull* 1995; **117**: 87–103.

Maloney D. Toxicity tests in animals: extrapolating to human risks. *Environmental Health Perspectives* 1993; **101**(5): 396–400.

Mansbach RS, Geyer MA. Blockade of potentiated startle in rats by 5-hydroxytryptamine receptor ligands. *Eur J Pharmacol* 1988; **156**:375–383.

Martin LJ, Sisoda SS, Koo EH, Cork LC, Dellovade TL, Weidemann A, Beyreuther K, Masters C, Price DL., Amyloid precursor protein in aged human primates. *Proc Natl Acad Sci USA* 1991; **88**: 1461–1465.

Millenson JR and Leslie J. The conditioned emotional response (CER) as a baseline for the study of antianxiety drugs. *Neuropharmacol.* 1974; **13**: 1–9.

Mineka S, Zinbarg R. Conditioning and ethological models of anxiety disorders: stress-in-dynamic-context anxiety models. *Nebr Symp Motiv* 1996; **43**: 135–210.

Monro A, Mehta D. Are single-dose toxicology studies in animals adequate to support single doses of a new drug in humans. *Clin Pharmacol Ther* 1996; **59** (3): 258–264.

Moore NA, Tye NC, Axton MS, Risius FC. The behavioral pharmacology of olanzapine, a novel 'atypical' antipsychotic agent. *J Pharmacol Exp Ther* 1992; **262**: 545–551.

Moreau JL, Bos M, Jenck F, Martin JR, Mortas P, Wichmann J. $5HT_{2c}$ receptor agonist exhibit antidepressant-like properties in the anhedonia model of depression in rats. *Eur Neuropsychopharmacol* 1996; **6**: 169–175.

Morgan M. Negative reinforcement. In: Weiskrantz L, ed. *Analysis of Behavioral Change*, Harper and Row, New York 1990: 19–49.

Mouradain MM, Chase TN. Gene therapy for Parkinson's disease: current knowledge and future perspective [editorial]. *Gene Ther* 1997; **4**: 504–506.

Nelson SD, Harvison PJ. Roles of cytochrome P450 in chemically induced cytotoxicity. In: Guengerich FP, ed. *Mammalian cytochromes P-450.* Florida: CRC Press, 1987, p. 19.

Ogawa S, Okuyama S, Araki H, Nakazato A, Otomo S. A rat model of phencylcidine psychosis. *Life Sciences* 1994; **55**: 1605–10.

Overstreet DH, and Janowsky DS. A cholinergic supersenstivity model of depression. In: Boulton A, Baker G, Martin-Iverson M, eds. *Neuromethods, Vol 19: Animal Models in Psychiatry.* Humana Press: Clifton, New Jersey, 1991, p. 81–114.

Overstreet DH, Russell RW, Crocker D, Gillin JC, and Janowsky DS. Genetic and pharmacological models of cholinergic supersensitivity and affective disorders. *Experientia* 1988; **44**: 465–472.

Overstreet DH, Russell RWW, Helps SC, Messenger M. Selective breeding for sensitivity to the anticholinesterase, DFP. *Psychopharmacol* 1979; **65**: 15–20.

Peck CC, Barr WH, Benet LZ, et al. Opportunities for integration of pharmacokinetics, pharmacodynamics, and toxicokinetics in rational drug development. *Clin Pharm Ther* 1992; **51**: 465–473.

Pellow P, File SE. Anxiolytic and anxiogenic drug effects on exploratory activity in an elevated plus maze: a novel test for anxiety in the rat. *Pharmacol Biochem Behav* 1986; **24**: 525–529.

Physician's Desk Reference. 51st edition. Montvale, Medical Economics Co., 1997. *Psychopharmacology* 1993; **110**: 479–489.

Randrup A, Munkvad I. Special antagonism of amphetamine-induced abnormal behavior. *Psychopharmacologia* 1965; **7**: 416-422.

Rapp PR, Amaral DG. Evidence for task-dependant memory dysfunction in the aged monkey. *J Neurosci* 1989; **9**: 3568–3576.

Reines SA. Early clinical trials in Alzheimer's disease: selection and evaluation of drug candidates. *Prog Clin Biol Res* 1989; **317**: 1283–1290.

Richardson JS. The olfactory bulbectomized rat as a model of major depressive disorder. In: Boulton A, Baker G, Martin-Iverson M, eds. *Neuromethods, Vol 19: Animal Models in Psychiatry.* Humana Press: Clifton, New Jersey, 1991, p. 61–79.

Rogers RJ, Cutler MG, Jackson JE. Behavioural effects in mice of subchronic buspirone, ondansetron, and tianeptine. II. The elevated plus-maze. *Pharmacol Biochem Behav* 1997; **56**: 295–303.

Sanger DJ, Joly D. Anxiolytic drugs and the acquisition of conditioned fear in mice. *Psychopharmacol* 1985; **85**: 284–288.

Sanger DJ, Joly D. Performance of a passive avoidance response is disrupted by compounds acting at the 5-HT$_{1A}$ receptors. *Behav Pharmacol* 1990; **1**: 235–240.

Sanger DJ. Animal models of anxiety and the screening of novel anxiolytic drugs. In Boulton A, Baker G, Martin-Iverson M, eds. *Neuromethods, Vol 19: Animal models in psychiatry.* Humana Press, Clifton New Jersey, 1991.

Sanger DJ. The effects of buspirone and related compounds on supressed operant responding in rats. J Pharmacol Exp Ther 1990; **254**: 420–426.

Scales MDC, Mahoney K. Animal toxicology studies on new medicines and their relationship to clinical exposure: a review of international recommendations. *Adverse Drug React Toxicol Rev* 1991; **10**: 155–68.

Schmajuk NA, Tyberg M. The hippocampal lesion model of schizophrenia. In: Boulton A, Baker G, Martin-Iverson M eds, *Neuromethods, vol 18: Animal models in psychiatry.* Humana Press: Clifton, New Jersey, 1991, p. 67–102.

Shanks N, Anisman H. Strain-specific effects of antidepressants on escape deficits induced by inescapable shock. *Pschopharmacol* 1989; **99**: 122–128.

Siglin JC, Rutledge GM. Laboratory Animal Management. In: Derelanko MJ, Hollinger MA, eds. *CRC Handbook of Toxicology.* Boca Raton: CRC Press, 1995, p. 1–50.

Smith G. Animal models of Alzheimer's disease: experimental cholinergic denervation. *Brain Res Rev* 1988; **13**: 103–118.

Spilker B. *Guide to Clinical Trials.* Raven Press, New York, 1991.

Sramek JJ, Cutler NR, Kurtz NM, Murphy MF, Carta A. *Optimizing the development of antipsychotic drugs.* Wiley, Chichester, England, 1996.

Steinpreis RE. The behavioral and neurochemical effects of phencyclidine in humans and animals: some implications for modeling psychosis. *Behav Brain Res* 1996; **74**: 45–55.

Temlett JA, Quinn NP, Jenner PG, Marsenden CD, Pourcher E, Bonnet AM, Agid Y, Markstein R, LaTaste X. Antiparkinsonian activity of CY 208-243, a partial D1 dopamine receptor agonist, in MPTP-treated marmosets and patients with Parkinson's disease. *Mov Disord* 1989; **4**: 261–265.

Tephly TR, Burchell B. UDP-glucuronosyltransferases: a family of detoxifying enzymes. *Trends Pharmacol* 1990; **11**: 276.

van den Heuvel MJ, Clark DG, Fielder RJ, Koundakjian PP, Olier GJA, Pelling D, Tomlinson NJ, Walker AP. The international validation of a fixed-dose procedure as an alternative to the classical LD$_{50}$ test. *Food and Chem Toxicol* 1990; **28**: 469–482.

van den Heuvel MJ, Dayan AD, and Shillaker RO. Evaluation of the BTS approach to the testing of substances and preparations for their acute toxicity. *Human Toxicol* 1987; **6**(4): 279–291.

Van Vliet PW, de Jongh J. Biokinetics and biokinetic models in risk assessment. *Hum Exp Toxicol* 1996; **15**: 799–809.

Vogel JR, Beer B, Clody DE. A simple and reliable conflict procedure for testing antianxiety agents. *Psychopharmacologia* 1971; **21**:1–7.

Voisin EM, Ruthsatz M, Collins JM, Hoyle PC. Extrapolation of animal toxicity to humans: interspecies comparisons in drug development. *Reg Toxicol Pharmacol* 1990; **12**: 107–116.

Weiner I, Shadach E, Tarrasch R, Kidron R, Feldon J. The latent inhibition model of schizophrenia: further validation using the atypical neuroleptic, clozapine. *Biol Psychiatry* 1996; **40**: 834–843.

Wesnes KA, Simpson PM. Can scopolamine produce a model of the memory deficits seen in aging and dementia? In: Gruneberg, MM, Morris PE, Sykes RN eds. *Practical aspects of memory: current research and issues.* Chichester: Wiley 1988, p. 1–6.

Willner P. Animal models of depression: validity and applications. In: Gessa G, Fratta W, Pani L, Serra G eds. *Depression and mania: from neurobiology to treatment.* New York: Raven Press, 1995, p. 19–41.

Yam J, Reer PJ, Bruce RD. Comparison of the up-and-down method and the fixed-dose procedure for acute oral toxicity testing. *Fd Chem Toxic* 1991; **29**(4): 259–263.

3   Surrogate endpoints

A common problem in drug development for many CNS indications is the lack of reliable and easily quantifiable outcome variables. As clinical assessments have sometimes been associated with low reliability and objectivity, researchers have pursued the development of biological markers of drug activity, or 'surrogate endpoints,' as secondary variables.

In order to be useful, however, a surrogate endpoint must meet several criteria. The surrogate response should be theoretically related to clinical improvement (e.g., through alterations of specific neurotransmitter systems that are implicated in the disease process). The surrogate endpoint should also correlate with or predict meaningful change in the primary clinical endpoint, with demonstrable validity in previous studies. Prentice (1989) has noted that a true surrogate endpoint will also 'yield a valid test of the null hypothesis of no association between treatment and the true response.' Additionally, if surrogate markers are to accelerate drug development, they must be quantifiable (with precision and reproducibility), reasonably inexpensive, and easily accessible (Cutler et al., 1994).

Although numerous biochemical, neurophysiological, pharmaco-dynamic, and neuroendocrine markers have been proposed in CNS clinical research, many have proven to be disappointing. There are several potential reasons for the failure of a surrogate endpoint. For example, the disease process could involve several causal pathways which do not all affect the surrogate marker. Thus, drug treatment could influence clinical outcome through pathways that are independent of the surrogate, underestimating the potential therapeutic value of the compound. Alternatively, drug treatment could affect only the pathway which involves the surrogate marker, which could overestimate the compound's efficacy (Fleming and DeMets, 1996). As the pathophysiology of many CNS disorders is not thoroughly understood, the determination of appropriate surrogate markers has understandably been a challenging prospect.

However, although these measures may not consistently correlate with therapeutic response, many have provided insight into the mechanism of action of novel compounds. Though the following examples demonstrate the difficulty of identifying valid and reliable surrogate endpoints, they also show the progress that has been made toward understanding the complexity of many CNS disorders.

EXAMPLES OF SURROGATE ENDPOINTS

Biochemical Markers

Depression: Monoamines and Their Metabolites

There is extensive evidence that monoaminergic, particularly serotonergic, abnormalities are involved in the pathogenesis of depression. Several studies have noted a reduction in brain concentrations of serotonin (5-HT) and alterations in serotonergic receptor function in depressed patients (reviewed in Grahame-Smith, 1989; Quintana, 1992; Sheline et al., 1995). Furthermore, patients who received antidepressants and underwent remission were shown to relapse upon depletion of 5-HT (Delgado et al., 1991). Finally, virtually all antidepressant compounds have been shown to enhance serotonergic transmission via direct or indirect mechanisms. Thus, several attempts have been made to characterize the effects of antidepressants on serotonin and its metabolites.

Antidepressants have previously been shown to increase platelet and plasma levels of 5-HT in patients with depression. Quintana (1992) reported that the administration of imipramine to 25 unmedicated depressed patients resulted in an increase in platelet 5-HT to the level of healthy control subjects. Another study reported that clomipramine administration resulted in an initial increase in plasma 5-HT which correlated with clinical improvement on the Montgomery-Asberg Depression Rating Scale (MADRS) over the 14-day treatment period (Spreux-Varoquaux et al., 1996). Similarly, long-term treatment with the antidepressant tianeptine resulted in an increase in plasma 5-HT concentrations in depressed patients which correlated with improvement on the MADRS (Ortiz et al., 1993). Celada et al. (1992) found that the monoamine oxidase inhibitors phenelzine and brofaromine both independently induced an increase in plasma 5-HT in depressed patients, with a significant inverse relationship between plasma 5-HT levels and Hamilton Rating Scale for Depression (HAM-D) scores.

Monoamine metabolite levels have also shown consistent effects in response to antidepressant treatment. Much of the research in this area has been conducted with monoamine oxidase inhibitors. In a double-blind study of moclobemide, depressed patients demonstrated dose-dependent reductions of plasma 3-methoxy-4-hydroxyphenylglycol (MHPG; a metabolite of norepinephrine) and homovanillic acid (HVA; a metabolite of dopamine) which correlated with improvements on the HAM-D (Markianos et al., 1994). Another study found that moclobemide administration resulted in a reduction in urinary excretion of MHPG; however, this reduction was not correlated with clinical improvement (Stefanis et al., 1988). Moclobemide was also reported to significantly reduce plasma concentrations of DHPH (a metabolite of norepinephrine), L-Dopa (a dopamine precursor), and HVA, although the initial changes in these biochemical markers also did not predict clinical outcome on the MADRS (Radat and Morand, 1996). Interestingly, plasma levels of 5-HIAA were unaffected in these studies.

As there is strong evidence that biochemical measures in CSF can reflect functional changes in the brain (Goodwin and Post, 1977), central measures of monoamine metabolites have also been evaluated as surrogate markers of antidepressant function. Although CSF measures require procedures that are not practical for large trials, their use in smaller, prospective studies could provide information beneficial to a drug development program.

The suppression of monoamine metabolite levels in CSF does not appear to be specific despite the pharmacological selectivity of many antidepressant compounds. For example, the norepinephrine uptake inhibitor desipramine and the 5-HT uptake inhibitor zimelidine both reduced CSF 5-HIAA as well as MHPG in depressed patients (Potter et al., 1985; Bertilsson et al., 1980). In a recent study by Sheline et al. (1997), 24 patients diagnosed with major depression received six weeks of treatment with either fluvoxamine or fluoxetine. CSF samples were collected after a 7–14 day placebo washout period prior to the study (baseline), and at the end of treatment. Both antidepressant compounds resulted in significant reductions of CSF 5-HIAA (57%), MHPG (48%), and HVA (17%). DeBellis et al. (1993) reported similar results in a study comparing CSF monoamine metabolite levels in nine depressed patients receiving fluoxetine. In these patients, CSF 5-HIAA and MHPG showed significant reductions following at least four weeks of treatment. Furthermore, these changes were concurrent with significant improvement on the HAM-D.

In another study evaluating the effects of clomipramine on CSF monoamine metabolite levels (Martensson et al., 1991), 12 patients with major depression demonstrated significant reductions in CSF 5-HIAA and MHPG following three weeks of treatment. Unfortunately, reductions of the metabolites were not clearly correlated with clinical improvement. Other evidence suggests that drug-induced changes in different neurotransmitter systems result in differential effects on behavior and emotion. Katz et al. (1994) evaluated 104 patients with unipolar or bipolar depression receiving treatment with tricyclic antidepressants, and found that reductions in CSF 5-HT metabolites were correlated with changes in mood (particularly anxiety and depressed mood) while reductions in norepinephrine metabolites were associated with changes in psychomotor activity.

As the pathology of depression appears to involve several neurotransmitter systems, some researchers have speculated that the relationship between monoamine metabolite levels may be a more significant factor. In an early retrospective study, Hsiao et al. (1987) examined CSF monoamine metabolite levels in depressed patients before and after antidepressant treatment. Patients were classified as responders if they had a HAM-D score lower than 10 with a drop in the HAM-D of 50% or more from pre-treatment to post-treatment, or a Bunney-Hamburg Depression Rating Scale (BDRS) score of 1 or 2 with a drop in score of 50% or more. While the absolute concentrations of CSF monoamine metabolites such as HVA, 5-HIAA, and MHPG did not differ between responders and non-responders before or after treatment, correlations between these metabolites differed significantly between the two groups. In responders to antidepressant treatment, treatment-induced changes in all three metabolites were found to correlate positively with each other. In non-responders, however, no correlations could be found at any time. However, as this study was retrospective, it is unclear if the relationship between the three metabolites could be used to predict treatment response in future studies.

Changes in CSF monoamines may represent the best biochemical surrogate endpoints for antidepressants at this time. Substantial progress has been made in the understanding of the mechanism of action of antidepressant compounds, largely due to the continued study of these biochemical markers. Although their predictive or correlative value is equivocal, these measures do provide valuable information on the pathways affected by various antidepressants which could be useful in the early development of novel compounds, as confirmation of a putative central mechanism of action.

Schizophrenia: Homovanillic Acid

Following the proposal of the dopamine hypothesis of schizophrenia, HVA has emerged as a potential biochemical surrogate marker of antipsychotic function. HVA assessments have been included in several studies of schizophrenic patients as an indirect measure of dopamine turnover. Previous evidence suggests that drug-free schizophrenic patients have higher total mean plasma levels of HVA than healthy control subjects (Lindstrom, 1985; Garcia et al., 1989). Additionally, several studies have reported a correlation between antipsychotic treatment response and a reduction in HVA levels.

In a study by Nagaoka et al. (1997), schizophrenic patients demonstrated a reduction in plasma HVA levels following the administration of haloperidol which correlated with improvement on the Brief Psychiatric Rating Scale (BPRS). Mazure et al. (1991) found similar results in patients receiving perphenazine, with changes in plasma HVA levels correlating with favorable clinical response. Another study reported time-dependent reductions in plasma HVA with neuroleptic treatment, and subsequent increases in HVA levels with neuroleptic withdrawal (Pickar et al., 1986). Longitudinal plasma measurements of HVA in this study were also highly correlated with psychosis ratings.

The effect of antipsychotic treatment on HVA levels has also been demonstrated with atypical antipsychotic compounds. In a study of eight treatment-resistant or treatment-intolerant schizophrenic patients, Green et al. (1993) reported that clozapine administration resulted in a reduction of plasma HVA during the initial weeks of treatment in responders, but not in non-responders. Another study reported a trend toward plasma HVA reductions in treatment-refractory schizophrenic patients demonstrating a clinical response to clozapine, although this effect did not reach significance (Davidson et al., 1993). Schizophrenic patients receiving sulpiride treatment also demonstrated a correlation between good clinical response and an overall reduction in plasma HVA levels after six weeks of treatment, although no relationship between psychotic ratings and HVA levels was noted during the treatment period (Alfredsson and Wiesel, 1990).

However, other studies have suggested that a biphasic HVA response is associated with antipsychotic response. For example, elevations in HVA during the first week of neuroleptic treatment, followed by a reduction back to baseline levels, have also demonstrated correlations with treatment response (Bowers et al., 1984; Scatton et al., 1982). In a study of schizophrenic patients receiving haloperidol for four weeks, Davila et al.

(1988) found that patients who demonstrated an elevation in HVA on day 4 *or* a reduction from days 4–28 showed the greatest improvement on the BPRS at the end of the study. These results suggest that an early increase followed by a steady reduction of plasma HVA was associated with a better clinical outcome. This biphasic response could be explained by antipsychotic antagonism at post-synaptic dopamine receptors, which would initially result in increased levels of circulating dopamine, followed by a longer term reduction of dopaminergic transmission.

However, these results are potentially clouded by the significant contribution of the peripheral nervous system to plasma levels of HVA (Pickar et al, 1988). To avoid this complication, some studies have included inhibitors of peripheral HVA production, such as debrisoquin. In an early study, Kendler et al. (1981) noted that debrisoquin pre-treatment did not effect haloperidol-induced changes in HVA, suggesting that the effects of neuroleptics on plasma HVA are due to central rather than peripheral mechanisms. Konicki et al. (1991) also reported that fluphenazine significantly increased 24-hour plasma HVA levels with or without the concurrent administration of debrisoquin. Duncan et al. (1993) evaluated schizophrenic patients pre-treated with debrisoquin with similar results, noting a biphasic response of plasma HVA associated with neuroleptic treatment. Patient responders demonstrated an increase in HVA 24 hours after the first dose, with a subsequent return to baseline levels. These studies provide support for the use of plasma HVA as a measure of CNS dopaminergic activity.

Although the underlying association between plasma HVA changes and central dopaminergic action is not completely clear, it appears that HVA measures are of some value in the prediction of clinical treatment response. However, the use of plasma HVA as a surrogate endpoint is not widespread at this time, due to the difficulty of the assay.

Neurophysiological Markers

Depression: Sleep EEG

Abnormal sleep patterns are an almost universal characteristic of depressed patients, and the suppression of REM sleep appears to be a effect common to several classes of antidepressant compounds. Sleep abnormalities typically observed in depression include an early onset of REM sleep, prolonged REM sleep, and a reduction of slow-wave sleep

(Mendlewicz and Kerkhofs, 1991; Thase et al., 1995; Hubain et al., 1995). The relationship between depression and sleep is not surprising, as the involvement of the serotonergic system in both states is well documented (reviewed in Leonard, 1996). Thus, EEG measures during sleep have become a potential neurophysiological surrogate endpoint of antidepressant response.

A large body of evidence suggests that all classes of antidepressant compounds affect sleep EEG patterns, and the most consistent of these effects is the suppression of REM sleep. In a study of paroxetine and amitriptyline in patients with major depression, both compounds resulted in a reduction of REM sleep, although side effect profiles differed (Staner et al., 1995). Buysse et al. (1996) reported that nortriptyline administration persistently decreased REM sleep in elderly depressed patients. Trazodone was also found to increase REM sleep latency and to significantly suppress REM sleep in patients with major depression (van Bemmel et al., 1992).

However, not all studies have reported consistent results. A study by Nofzinger et al. (1995) was the first report of an antidepressant compound which shortened REM latency and increased REM sleep. A total of 18 male depressed patients receiving bupropion (n = 7) or fluoxetine (n = 11) underwent an all-night sleep EEG study before treatment and after partial or full remission. The administration of bupropion to depressed male patients resulted in an increase in percent REM sleep and total REM time, in direct contrast to the results observed with fluoxetine. Nefazodone has also been shown to significantly increase REM sleep time, although no reductions of REM latency have been observed with this compound (Sharpley et al., 1992). In another double-blind trial, Sonntag et al. (1996) compared the effects of the tricyclic antidepressants trimipramine and imipramine on sleep EEG patterns in male inpatients with major depression. Both of these treatments resulted in significant clinical improvement of depressive symptoms, although they demonstrated different neurophysiological profiles. While imipramine exhibited the 'classical' antidepressant suppression of REM sleep, trimipramine actually enhanced REM sleep.

Furthermore, suppression of REM sleep has not always correlated with improvement in depressive symptomatology, which casts doubt on the utility of this measure as a surrogate endpoint measure. For example, in a study comparing alprazolam and amitriptyline in the treatment of major depressive disorder, Hubain et al. (1990) reported that these compounds displayed similar effects on EEG, such as a shortening of REM sleep. However, amitriptyline was significantly more effective than alprazolam according to HAM-D measures, with a large number of patients discontinuing alprazolam treatment due to ineffectiveness against depressive symptoms. Thus, while EEG measures can confirm the central serotonergic activity of an antidepressant compound, this neurophysiological evaluation may not predict meaningful clinical response and is therefore a poor surrogate endpoint.

Alzheimer's Disease: EEG

There is strong evidence that the cholinergic system plays a role in modulating EEG function (Abe et al., 1997; Bjorklund et al., 1996), and that EEG slowing is pervasive characteristic of Alzheimer's disease (AD) (Lopez et al., 1997; Elmstahl et al., 1994; Prichep et al., 1994). Moreover, EEG measures have been shown to correlate with cognitive and functional decline in patients with AD. In a study by Schreiter-Gasser et al. (1994) in 15 presenile AD patients, the degree of dementia was strongly reflected by an increase in power in the delta (slow-wave) frequency band of the EEG. In another study, quantitative EEG measures correlated with the severity of cognitive impairment in patients in different stages of AD (Passero et al., 1995). Primavera et al. (1990) also reported a statistically significant correlation between MMSE scores and quantitative EEG measures in AD patients and healthy elderly subjects.

Preclinical studies have indicated that lesions of the basal forebrain reduce power in the beta frequencies with concurrent impairments in memory (Abe et al., 1997), suggesting that EEG slowing in AD could be the result of reduced cholinergic input to the cortex. Thus, compounds that enhance cholinergic transmission, such as acetylcholinesterase inhibitors, would be expected to normalize EEG function. In fact, several studies have reported EEG enhancement with compounds for AD. In one such study, Shigeta et al. (1993) evaluated three patients with mild AD receiving long-term treatment with tacrine at doses between 40 and 160 mg. At high doses of tacrine, patients demonstrated a marked increase in the mean EEG frequency in frontal, temporal, and parieto-occipital regions of the brain. Another study also reported an improvement of EEG function in 10 AD patients following the intravenous administration of physostigmine (Gustafson, 1993).

Of course, the utility of EEG function as a surrogate endpoint for AD compounds also requires that this measure correlate with clinical improvement. There have been few studies in this area, although the results have largely been positive. In a quantitative EEG study by Perryman and Fitten (1991), the baseline dominant parietal rhythms of patients with AD were significantly different from controls, and the severity of cognitive impairment was related to the degree of parietal slowing. Following treatment with tacrine, three patients demonstrated significant improvement on cognitive measures, two of which also demonstrated enhanced parietal EEG rhythms. More robust results were reported in a single-dose pharmaco-EEG study of tacrine in 14 patients with AD and seven age-matched controls (Alhainen et al., 1991). All subjects received a single, 50 mg oral dose of tacrine 90 minutes prior to an EEG recording. Following seven weeks of tacrine treatment, six of the 14 AD patients were designated as responders, based on MMSE evaluations. EEG frequency analysis revealed that the responders had demonstrated a significant increase in the alpha to theta ratio in comparison to non-responders or control subjects. Thus, this relative change was a sensitive discriminator of responders from non-responders to treatment.

In another, double-blind, crossover study of tacrine (Minthon et al., 1993), 17 patients with AD received each of three six-week treatment regimens: tacrine and lecithin, tacrine and placebo, and placebo. Patients were evaluated with clinical ratings, psychometric testing, and EEG measures. At the end of the study, six patients had improved (responders), five patients demonstrated no change (non-responders), and six patients had deteriorated (non-responders). Among the patient responders, EEG measures showed more high frequency activity.

Thus, the above studies suggest that treatment with an acetyl-cholinesterase inhibitor results in an enhancement of EEG, which correlates with improvement on clinical evaluations. Although not practical for large studies, EEG evaluations could be included in early studies as a surrogate measure to confirm central activity.

Pharmacodynamic Markers

Depression: Platelet 5-HT receptors

Although the relative involvement of various serotonergic receptor subtypes in the pathology of depression is unclear at this time, there is some evidence that increased $5\text{-}HT_2$ receptor density might be a significant factor. $5\text{-}HT_2$ receptor binding studies have suggested that chronic antidepressant treatment decreases $5\text{-}HT_2$ receptor number and function (Zemlan and Garver, 1990). In addition, novel antidepressants with $5\text{-}HT_2$ antagonist properties, such as nefazodone, have demonstrated efficacy against depressive symptoms (Rickels et al., 1995; Fontaine et al., 1994).

As central serotonergic receptor density is not easily measured, platelet receptors constitute a more easily accessible peripheral surrogate marker. Previous studies have noted differences in platelet 5-HT_2 receptor densities between depressed patients and healthy controls. For example, Sheline et al. (1995) collected platelets from 35 depressed outpatients and 14 control subjects following a minimum three week drug free period, and found that platelet 5-HT_2 receptor density values were higher in depressed patients than in controls. Furthermore, a trend towards a positive correlation between cognitive depressive symptoms (as assessed on the HAM-D) and the 5-HT_2 receptor density values was also evident. In another study of 25 medication-free patients with major depression and 20 healthy controls, Hrdina et al. (1995) evaluated the density and affinity of 5-HT_2 receptors labeled with radioactive LSD. The B_{max} of platelet 5-HT_2 receptors was found to be significantly (52%) greater in depressed patients than in controls.

There is also support for an association between platelet 5-HT_2 receptor densities and suicidality in depressed patients. Bakish et al. (1997) reported a strong correlation between the HAM-D suicidality item and an increased platelet 5-HT_2 receptor density in 21 depressed patients. A prospective study of 131 hospitalized psychiatric patients and 40 healthy controls reported that the mean B_{max} of platelet 5-HT_{2A} receptors for patients who met HAM-D criteria for suicidal behavior was significantly higher than for nonsuicidal patients or healthy controls (Pandey et al., 1995). Biegon et al. (1990a) evaluated platelet 5-HT_2 receptors in 22 suicidal and 19 healthy male subjects, using tritiated ketanserin. The results indicated that mean receptor binding in the suicidal patients was significantly (50%) higher than in controls.

More importantly, platelet 5-HT_2 receptor densities have demonstrated alterations in response to antidepressant treatment. For example, Biegon et al. (1990b) evaluated platelet 5-HT_2 receptors in 15 patients with major depression during a drug-free state and following one and three weeks of treatment with the antidepressant maprotiline. Alterations in receptor binding correlated with clinical changes on the Beck and HAM-D rating scales; clinical improvement was associated with reduction in 5-HT_2 binding. In those patients who did not demonstrate clinical change or who worsened during the treatment period, 5-HT_2 receptor binding remained unchanged or increased, respectively. In addition, Stahl et al. (1993) reported that downregulation of 5-HT_2 receptors, as assessed by platelet shape-change responses, was associated with clinical response in depressed patients treated with nortriptyline. Although few studies have utilized platelet receptor density as a surrogate endpoint at this time, some researchers have supported its use as an index of antidepressant efficacy (Bakish et al., 1997; Biegon et al., 1990b).

Alzheimer's Disease: Acetylcholinesterase Inhibition

One of the most successful pharmacological strategies in the treatment of AD involves the inhibition of acetylcholinesterase (AChE), an enzyme which hydrolyzes and inactivates acetylcholine. Several compounds of this class have shown efficacy in patients with AD, including tacrine (Knapp et al., 1994), SDZ ENA 713 (Anand and Hartman, 1996), eptastigmine (Canal and Imbimbo, 1996), and velnacrine (Antuono, 1995). This strategy has also provided researchers with a rational surrogate endpoint, as assays of AChE activity in plasma or CSF are currently available. However, the assessment of acetylcholinesterase inhibitors using measures of AChE activity is complicated by several factors.

There are two types of cholinesterase, 'true' or 'specific' (AChE) and 'pseudo' or 'non-specific' (butyrylcholinesterase, or BChE) (Lawson and Barr, 1987). These two cholinesterase types are present in varying concentrations in CSF and blood, and are affected differently by various acetylcholinesterase inhibitors. AChE is a much more accurate index of neurotoxicity, and is the main target of most AD compounds (Sanz et al., 1991). However, BChE levels in plasma are approximately 1000 times greater than AChE levels (St. Clair et al., 1986), and a measure of total plasma cholinesterase will largely reflect BChE activity. Because many compounds differentially affect the two cholinesterase types, it is often necessary to isolate the drug's effect on AChE. Thus, many studies evaluate red blood cell (RBC) cholinesterase, which largely consists of AChE (Sirviö et al., 1989; Barr et al., 1988), and/or will include a compound to selectively suppress the activity of BChE, such as tetraisopropyl-pyrophosphoramide (iso-OMPA), in samples of blood or CSF prior to analysis.

There is also little BChE activity in CSF, which is perhaps the most direct means of measuring central AChE inhibition (Hallack and Giacobini, 1989). Previous studies have revealed that the evaluation of neuro-transmitters and synthetic/degradative enzymes in CSF provide a reliable index of central neuronal activity in man (Cutler et al., 1985; Polinsky et al., 1989). We recently conducted a single-center, open-label, multiple-dose study to evaluate the effects of an acetylcholinesterase inhibitor on AChE and BChE activity in CSF, and to correlate these parameters with pharmacokinetic measures. In addition, the cognitive effects of this compound were assessed using the Computerized Neuropsychological Test Battery (CNTB).

A total of 18 patients (9 males, 9 females; mean age 62.6 years) meeting NINCDS-ADRDA criteria for probable AD participated in this study in six sequential groups of three patients each. Patients were titrated from an initial dose of 1 mg bid to one of six target doses (1, 2, 3, 4, 5, or 6 mg bid) in 1 mg bid/week increments. After patients had been maintained at their target dose for at least three days, continuous CSF samples were obtained via an indwelling lumbar catheter beginning within 0.5 hours prior to and for 12 hours following the final dose. CSF AChE and BChE activity were assayed using the method of Ellman et al. (1961).

Administration of the study compound resulted in significant dose-dependent inhibition of CSF AChE ($p < 0.05$), with a maximum mean inhibition of 62% in the 6 mg bid treatment group. Significant inhibition of CSF BChE was also observed ($p < 0.05$), although this inhibition was highly variable over the time points evaluated. Overall, the compound was well tolerated in this population at doses up to 6 mg bid. Improvement on the CNTB was observed for patients receiving higher doses of the compound, and a significant correlation was observed between the improvement on the CNTB summary score from baseline to the post-dose evaluation and the inhibition of AChE and BChE in CSF. Thus, the rapid, sustained, dose-dependent inhibition of CSF AChE, attended by cognitive enhancement, suggests that the compound has the potential to produce a meaningful therapeutic benefit in AD patients. This study is discussed in greater detail in Chapter 5.

Although the evaluation of CSF provides the most direct measure of central AChE activity, the lumbar procedure with continuous sampling is likely to be too complex and impractical for large clinical trials. Thus, this measure is best employed in smaller numbers of patients, as in the bridging study (see Chapter 5 for a discussion of bridging methodology). AChE assessment in blood, however, is easily accessible and could provide a valuable peripheral surrogate marker of central cholinergic activity.

At this time, the relationship between central and peripheral AChE activity remains somewhat controversial. In early animal studies, Hallack and Giacobini (1987) found a strong linear correlation ($r = 0.98$) between cholinesterase activity in rat brain tissue and in both plasma and erythrocytes following the intramuscular administration of physostigmine. The route of administration was found to be an important factor, as blood cholinesterase inhibition was a reliable marker 10–20 minutes after intravenous physostigmine, and 30–60 minutes following an oral dose (Hallack and Giacobini, 1989). The inhibition of cholinesterase following the administration of metrifonate followed a different time course in blood than in brain; cholinesterase inhibition in erythrocytes and plasma was greater than inhibition in brain during the first 60 minutes. However, cholinesterase was inhibited in the same proportion in brain, plasma, and erythrocytes after the initial 60 minutes (Hallack and Giacobini, 1989). Cholinesterase inhibition in plasma was also found to be a relatively accurate predictor of cholinesterase inhibition in the brain following the administration of tacrine (Hallack and Giacobini, 1989).

Similar results were observed by Thomsen et al. (1991), who examined the effects of three different acetylcholinesterase inhibitors on AChE activity in human brain and blood samples. Samples were obtained from postmortem brain tissue from 11 individuals, in addition to samples of brain tissue and blood from four subjects who had cortical material removed to gain access to tumors. During in vitro analysis of the samples, BChE activity was suppressed with iso-OMPA. Both physostigmine and tacrine resulted in AChE inhibition in erythrocytes that closely paralleled that in cortical tissue.

However, Thompson's group also reported that galanthamine inhibited AChE in erythrocytes ten times more potently than in brain tissue. Furthermore, novel acetylcholinesterase inhibitors, such as SDZ ENA 713, have been distinguished by a selective effect on CSF (brain) AChE rather than plasma, suggesting that the relationship between peripheral and central measures of inhibition could depend on the compound under investigation. Another potential complication with peripheral measures of AChE inhibition is that the pharmacokinetics of therapeutic compounds could differ substantially in the central compartment and in plasma.

Several clinical trials of acetylcholinesterase inhibitors have included plasma or erythrocyte measures of AChE in order to characterize the pharmacodynamic activity of the compound. Although there is no guideline for how much inhibition is necessary to achieve therapeutic benefit, some studies have successfully noted correlations between AChE measures and clinical improvement. In a large, multicenter, double-blind study of the novel acetylcholinesterase inhibitor donepezil (n = 141), patients received one of three doses of donepezil or placebo for 12 weeks (Rogers and Friedhoff, 1996). Clinical improvement was evaluated with the Alzheimer's Disease Assessment Scale cognitive subscale (ADAS-cog) and the MMSE. Red blood cell AChE activity was measured at baseline and at the end of study. Donepezil administration resulted in a maximum RBC AChE inhibition of 76–84%, and AChE inhibition was significantly correlated with the change in ADAS-cog scores (p = 0.008).

Another study by Canal and Imbimbo (1996) indicated that a high percentage of AChE inhibition does not appear to be necessary to achieve therapeutic efficacy. In their multicenter, double-blind, placebo-controlled study, 103 AD patients received eptastigmine (n = 83) or placebo (n = 20) for four weeks. A battery of clinical and cognitive assessments were administered at baseline and at the end of the study, including the Logical Memory Test, Semantic Word Fluency Test, Trail Making Test, Index of Independence in Activities of Daily Living (IADL), Instrumental Activities of Daily Living Scales, and the Physician and Caregiver Clinical Global Impression of Change (Physician CGIC). At steady state, eptastigmine administration resulted in an average daily AChE inhibition of 13–54%. A significantly higher percentage of patients receiving eptastigmine demonstrated improvement on the Physician CGIC and IADL than patients receiving placebo. In patients receiving eptastigmine, improvement on all cognitive tests and clinical scales demonstrated a U-shaped relationship with AChE inhibition, indicating that moderate inhibition was associated with the highest level of improvement.

There are clearly several factors which can affect the relationship between peripheral and central inhibition, including timing, characteristics of the particular compound under investigation (i.e., specificity for brain versus plasma AChE), and the mode of drug administration. Thus, we do not recommend reliance on blood AChE as a surrogate endpoint. However, with further study and refinement, this peripheral marker may become a reasonable index of central AChE inhibition, and future studies to this end are warranted.

Alzheimer's Disease: Salivary Amylase

We recently investigated a novel, potential peripheral marker in a study of the muscarinic agonist, xanomeline (Sramek et al., 1995a). Xanomeline has demonstrated a high affinity for M_1 muscarinic receptors in vitro and in vivo (Shannon et al., 1994); however, some lower-affinity binding at other muscarinic receptor subtypes may be unavoidable. While M_1 receptors are found in neural tissue, M_3 receptors are typically located in secretory organs, such as the pancreas and salivary glands. Activity at the M_3 receptor subtype results in an increase in intestinal and salivary secretions.

In our double-blind, placebo-controlled study, we measured serum amylase, fractionated into pancreatic and salivary isoenzymes, as a potential marker of M_3 receptor activity associated with the MTD of xanomeline tartrate. Two doses of xanomeline (100 and 115 mg, tid) were evaluated in 12 AD patients. There was a trend toward increased salivary amylase at the highest dose tested (Figure 3.1), although this effect did not achieve statistical significance (potentially due to the small sample size coupled with a higher

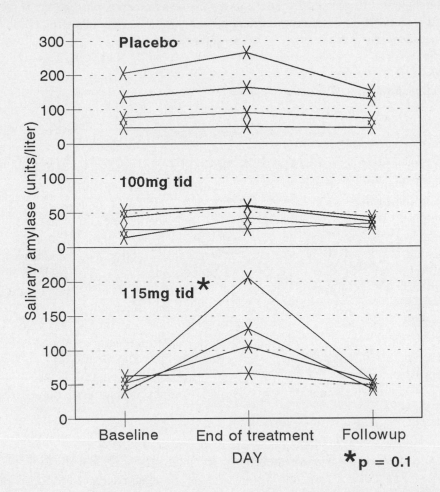

Figure 3.1 Effect of xanomeline on salivary amylase levels. Individual patients are represented.

baseline level in the placebo group). In one patient receiving 115 mg tid, salivary amylase levels increased to 400% over baseline, and were accompanied by moderate hypersalivation. This patient was discontinued from the study due to intolerable adverse events. No changes in pancreatic amylase were evident, although the reason for the lack of effect on pancreatic muscarinic receptors is unclear.

If we assume that elevations in salivary amylase are due to M_3-receptor mediated effects, it appears that the specificity for M_1 receptors might begin to disappear at higher doses. Thus, although these results are preliminary, we conclude that elevated salivary amylase may be associated with the lower end of the toxicological spectrum of xanomeline tartrate in patients with AD, and is a potentially useful marker of M_3 receptor activity.

Neuroendocrine Markers

Depression: The Dexamethasone Suppression Test

Overactivity of the hypothalamic-pituitary-adrenocortical (HPA) axis and hypercortisolism are two of the most consistent biological abnormalities observed in depressed patients (Carroll et al., 1976a; Poland et al., 1987; Rubin et al., 1987). Measures of such neuroendocrine abnormalities in depressed patients have become a potential 'window into the brain,' as plasma levels of these peptides reflect central activity, particularly in reference to 5-HT function (Levy and Van de Kar, 1992). The relationship between the serotonergic system and the HPA axis is well documented. Serotonergic neurons from the dorsal raphe and other nuclei innervating hypothalamic areas which control hormone secretion provide a physiological basis for the link between depression and neuroendocrine function. The study of neuroendocrine function and depression is also appealing because the neuropeptides affected in depression are also implicated in stress, a state which is often thought to precipitate depressive episodes.

One measure of cortisol function commonly used in studies of antidepressants is the dexamethasone suppression test (DST). Perhaps the most well-studied neuroendocrine assessment in psychiatry, this test enjoyed an extended period of popularity in the diagnosis and prognosis of depression. Briefly, the DST evaluates the suppression of various neuropeptides, including cortisol, in response to the administration of dexamethasone. While healthy subjects generally show substantial inhibition of neuropeptide release, a large body of evidence suggests that patients with depression demonstrate abnormal responses to the DST, including a failure to suppress cortisol release or a premature release from cortisol suppression (Carroll et al., 1976b; Carroll et al., 1981; Peselow et al., 1983). Due to a lack of specificity and an inability to distinguish between chronic and acute hypercortisolism, however, the DST fell from favor as a diagnostic marker (Aguilar et al., 1984; Stokes et al., 1984; Calloway et al., 1984). Although no longer used in the diagnosis of depression, the DST is still often included in trials of novel antidepressants as a surrogate endpoint measure.

The literature reveals mixed results regarding the ability of the DST to predict clinical response to antidepressant treatment. In one study, Heuser et al. (1996) evaluated the effects of amitriptyline in elderly depressed patients (n = 39) and healthy control subjects (n = 14) treated for six weeks. In comparison to the healthy controls, the depressed patients demonstrated a higher cortisol release in response to the DST prior to treatment; this abnormal response normalized within one week of amitriptyline administration. In another study by Alvarez et al. (1997), the DST was administered to 105 depressed patients following four weeks of antidepressant-lithium treatment. Patients who were DST non-suppressors at baseline were more likely to be responders; however, cortisol responses among these patients failed to normalize after treatment.

A failure to normalize DST suppression in response to antidepressant treatment is generally predictive of a poor prognosis. For example, in a study of elderly depressed outpatients, the DST was administered at baseline and after three and seven weeks of treatment with either nortriptyline or phenelzine (Rush et al., 1988). All patients who continued to demonstrate abnormal responses on the DST (n = 7) did not respond to antidepressant treatment. These findings were echoed in a meta-analysis conducted by Ribeiro et al. (1993). Based on 144 articles evaluating the DST as a predictive measure of outcome in depression, these authors reported that a persistent nonsuppression of cortisol on the DST was associated with a poor prognosis, including early relapse and a poor outcome after discharge.

However, other evidence suggests that the DST is not a good candidate for a surrogate endpoint in depression. First, several studies have noted that only approximately half of patients with depression are DST non-suppressors (Extein et al., 1985; Barry and Dinan, 1990; Twardowska and Rybakowski, 1996). While the majority of depressed patients demonstrate some kind of neuroendocrine abnormality, not all are revealed by the DST (Barry and Dinan, 1990). Secondly, some researchers have argued that there is no true correlation between DST response and therapeutic improvement. For example, Gibbons et al. (1987) argued that normalization of the DST after antidepressant treatment is not indicative of clinical response, but is instead due to a regression toward the mean. These authors evaluated two studies of depressed patients which reported a relationship between normalization of the DST and clinical improvement, and found that post-dexamethasone cortisol levels decreased regardless of clinical response to antidepressant treatment. In another study (Peselow et al., 1987), 127 outpatients with major depression were administered the DST during depression and after recovery. The value of the DST as a monitor or long-term outcome was not favorable, as many patients remained stable over a six month period regardless of abnormal cortisol values after recovery. Finally, there is no clear consensus on how antidepressants normalize HPA/cortisol function in patients with depression, which casts doubt upon the theoretical basis for neuroendocrine responses as a surrogate endpoint. Thus, currently available evidence suggests that the DST cannot be recommended as a surrogate endpoint measure of antidepressant function.

Depression: D-fenfluramine Challenge

D-fenfluramine, a serotonin-releasing agent, results in increased prolactin release, an effect that is blunted in depressed patients as compared to healthy controls (Lichtenberg et al., 1992; O'Keane and Dinan, 1991; Mitchell and Smythe, 1990). Responses to d-fenfluramine challenge also appear to be more severely blunted in depressed patients with a history of suicidality (Malone et al., 1996; Cleare et al., 1996). Thus, this neuroendocrine probe has been investigated as a surrogate measure in trials of antidepressants.

Although there is evidence that antidepressant treatment enhances the prolactin response to d-fenfluramine (O'Keane et al., 1992), no relationship with clinical response has been established at this time. One potential problem with this test as a surrogate marker is that the distinction between depressed patients and healthy controls may be dependent on the age of the subjects. Lerer et al. (1996) administered the d-fenfluramine challenge test to patients with major endogenous depression (n = 39) and healthy control subjects (n = 30), and reported that prolactin responses were significantly blunted in younger depressed patients as compared to controls, but not in older patients. Another study found a 38% lower maximum prolactin response to d-fenfluramine challenge in depressed patients ages 30 and under, as compared to age-matched healthy controls, while older depressed patients did not differ from older controls (Mann et al., 1995).

Thus, the prolactin response to d-fenfluramine challenge in depressed patients is incompletely understood at this time. Further study is necessary to evaluate the value of this measure as a surrogate endpoint in depression.

Schizophrenia: Prolactin

Elevations in prolactin levels result from D_2 receptor blockade in the tuberoinfundibular tract of the hypothalamus, and have been used as an index of central antidopaminergic activity. Indeed, many neuroleptics enhance prolactin secretion, and some attempts have been made to correlate increased prolactin secretion with greater dopaminergic antagonism, and perhaps efficacy in schizophrenic patients.

Previous evidence with typical antipsychotics has supported an association between prolactin levels and antipsychotic efficacy. For example, Pandurangi et al. (1989) reported a significant relationship between higher serum prolactin levels and treatment response to the antipsychotic molindone. Similarly, Bowers et al. (1987) found that greater prolactin levels at steady state were significantly related to global outcome in male patients treated with fixed daily doses of haloperidol for 10 days.

Neuroendocrine challenge tests have also indicated a link between prolactin responses and clinical efficacy. In a study of patients treated with clozapine, Lieberman et al. (1994) found that a greater inhibition of prolactin release in response to apomorphine stimulation was correlated with a better therapeutic outcome. Additionally, Curtis et al. (1995) noted that clozapine treatment resulted in an attenuation of prolactin secretion in response to d-fenfluramine challenge. Changes in symptom ratings correlated significantly with the reduction of prolactin response to the challenge.

Moreover, lower levels of prolactin following the administration of typical antipsychotics have been linked to the risk of relapse. In a one-year study of 29 schizophrenic outpatients, Faraone et al. (1986) found that mean serum prolactin levels two weeks after neuroleptic dose reduction were significantly lower among those patients that experienced relapse. Additionally, another study reported that although prolactin levels did not differ between patients who did or did not experience relapse, serum prolactin levels were lower before relapse episodes than before stable periods (Faraone et al., 1987).

However, other studies have failed to identify a relationship between prolactin levels and antipsychotic efficacy. In two studies of chlorpromazine, serum prolactin levels did not predict clinical response in schizophrenic patients (Meltzer and Busch, 1983; Meltzer et al., 1983). There also appears to be a ceiling effect for the prolactin response. For example, Seiler et al. (1994) noted that plasma levels of the neuroleptic benperidol as low as 2–3 nanograms were sufficient to deplete pituitary prolactin stores. Additionally, another study found that prolactin levels increased with doses of haloperidol up to 100 mg, but did not increase further with higher doses (Scatton et al., 1982).

Another problem with using prolactin as a surrogate endpoint of antipsychotic function is that not all antipsychotic compounds are potent D_2 receptor antagonists. The association between prolactin secretion and D_2 receptor binding has been confirmed using single photon emission computed tomography (SPECT). In a study of 12 male schizophrenic patients receiving haloperidol, benperidol, or clozapine, prolactin levels were positively correlated with D_2 receptor occupancy (Schlegel et al., 1996). Additionally, there is evidence that 'atypical' antipsychotic compounds, which are generally less potent at D_2 receptors, do not enhance the release of prolactin (Beasley et al., 1996; Lee et al., 1995; Wetzel et al., 1995). One exception is the atypical antipsychotic risperidone, which is a D_2 receptor antagonist that does induce an increase in prolactin secretion (Megens et al., 1994). Thus, although prolactin levels have the potential to correlate with clinical response to antipsychotic therapy, the value of this surrogate endpoint is dependent upon the pharmacodynamic profile of the compound, and cannot be used as a general measure.

Schizophrenia: Growth Hormone

Although less well-studied, growth hormone (GH) has also been evaluated as a potential surrogate endpoint in schizophrenia. GH secretion is stimulated by dopamine, and is mediated through agonist activity at post-synaptic dopaminergic receptors in the anterior pituitary (Wong et al., 1993; Chang et al., 1990). Thus, antipsychotic compounds which are dopamine antagonists inhibit the release of GH.

Medicated schizophrenic patients have demonstrated weaker GH responses to apomorphine pretreatment in comparison to healthy unmedicated subjects, potentially reflecting the antagonism of central post-synaptic dopamine receptors by neuroleptic treatment (Muller-Spahn et al., 1984; Scheinin et al., 1985). Additionally, one study found evidence of a relationship between high thought disorder scores and elevated GH responses to apomorphine in schizophrenic patients (Zemlan et al., 1986). Attempts to correlate GH measures with clinical response, however, are few at this time. One study designed to evaluate the effects of dose reduction in schizophrenic patients receiving haloperidol included blockade of bromocriptine-induced GH response as an index of central function (Hirschowitz et al., 1997). Future studies of antipsychotics which target specific dopamine receptors might help to clarify the value of GH as a marker of central antipsychotic activity. In particular, the effects of autoreceptor or partial dopamine agonists should prove interesting; preliminary results indicate that these compounds result in increases of GH (Wiedemann and Kellner, 1994).

Anxiety: Cortisol

Although the mechanism is unknown at this time, several anxiolytic compounds have been reported to increase levels of plasma cortisol. This effect appears to be specific to anxiolytics with $5\text{-}HT_{1A}$ receptor agonist properties, including the azapirones (Cowen et al., 1990), leading some researchers to speculate that the cortisol response is a index of 5-HT receptor function. Lesch et al. (1992) examined hormone responses to ipsapirone in patients with panic disorder (n = 14) and healthy controls (n = 14), and found that while ipsapirone induced cortisol release in both groups, the neuroendocrine response in patients was attenuated in comparison to controls. These authors concluded that the impaired cortisol response in patients was due to a subsensitivity of pre- and post-synaptic $5\text{-}HT_{1A}$ receptor systems in panic disorder. In contrast, Norman et al. (1994) reported no differences in cortisol responses to buspirone between patients with obsessive compulsive disorder (OCD) (n = 16) and healthy controls (n = 16), and suggested that dysfunction of the $5\text{-}HT_{1A}$ receptor is not present in OCD.

Although no attempts have been made to correlate the cortisol response to anxiolytic efficacy in humans, animal studies have not been encouraging. In a study of the $5\text{-}HT_{1A}$ receptor agonist flesinoxan, increased cortisol levels were not related to its anxiolytic effects in a shock-stress paradigm (Groenink et al., 1995). Furthermore, other classes of anxiolytic compounds, such as the benzodiazepines, have been shown to *reduce* cortisol levels in patients and healthy subjects (Abelson et al., 1996; Roy-Byrne et al., 1991; Lopez et al., 1990). Thus, this neuroendocrine marker is potentially useful as a measure of $5\text{-}HT_{1A}$ agonist activity; however, its utility as a surrogate endpoint does not appear promising at this time.

CONCLUSIONS ON EXAMPLES OF SURROGATE MARKERS

The above examples illustrate the challenge of identifying valid and reliable surrogate markers. While the concept of quantifiable, objective endpoints is appealing, the use of surrogate markers introduces the risk of finding clinically misleading results. However, in Phase I trials in the patient population, carefully selected surrogate endpoints based on a solid theoretical background can be valuable in the preliminary evaluation of a drug. Additionally, surrogate endpoints may be useful in the confirmation of a drug's central activity and mechanism of action, as long as there is rational basis for the belief that the endpoint will be predictive of efficacy in Phase II/III trials, where more definitive endpoints are required (Mamelok, 1994). The weight of the surrogate endpoint is also dependent upon the compound under investigation; a lack of effect on surrogate markers with a novel compound may be expected, while such a result with a 'me-too' compound might be taken more seriously as a sign of failure.

Perhaps the greatest difficulty of surrogate endpoints is the question of whether they reflect the actual clinical utility of the investigational compound. However, this problem leads to the larger issue of what defines the standard for clinical efficacy. Comparative trials in development, perhaps as early as Phase II, can be useful in making decisions regarding the clinical utility of a compound by comparison to a known standard.

HOW DO YOU CHOOSE THE CORRECT DOSE?

As discussed in Chapter 1, inaccurate or suboptimal dose selection for Phase II clinical trials can result in the delay or even discontinuation of a drug development program. An inaccurate dose range can lead to two distinct problems. If the dose range selected is too high, patient attrition due to a high incidence of adverse events could disrupt the progress of a clinical trial. Even more seriously, unacceptable toxicity could result in the discontinuation of a clinical development program. Alternatively, if the dose range selected is too low, potentially efficacious doses could be left untested. As the vast majority of CNS compounds have demonstrated a linear dose-response curve, efficacy is sometimes observed only at the higher end of the tolerable dose range; thus, a program could be abandoned for lack of therapeutic benefit if the minimum effective dose is not reached.

Early Dose-Finding Procedures

The first priority in selecting a dose range is safety. Phase I studies are designed to explore a compound's preliminary parameters of toxicity and to identify a well-tolerated dose range in healthy subjects. Previous preclinical research has demonstrated that a margin of exposure of $1/100^{th}$ of the No Observed Adverse Effect Level (NOAEL) in the most sensitive animal species provides adequate safety for testing initial dosage in human subjects (Newman et al., 1993). The dose is then escalated, usually on a semi-logarithmic basis, up to the minimum intolerated dose (MID). The MID can be defined as the dose at which 50% of patients experience severe or multiple moderate adverse events probably related to the study drug or one patient experiences a serious adverse event (defined as medically unacceptable) believed to be related to the study drug. The dose immediately below this one is the maximum tolerated dose (MTD). The MTD can then be used as a basis for dose-ranging studies, or 'bridging studies,' in patients early in Phase II.

The goal of a bridging study is to find a safe and effective dose of the drug for the target patient population (Cutler and Sramek 1995a; Cutler and Sramek, 1995b; Cutler et al., 1996). This goal can be achieved by demonstrating a dose-response relationship for adverse events. For the majority of CNS compounds, therapeutic efficacy improves with increasing dose up to a point at which the risks and discomforts of adverse events begin to outweigh any beneficial effects. Thus, well-designed bridging studies can identify the dose range at which beneficial effects are most likely to occur without prohibitive side effects. This dose range will then be employed in later Phase II trials, which attempt to determine whether or not a drug is efficacious and outline a range of side effects.

In smaller dose-ranging studies, surrogate markers can be useful as a preliminary index of central activity (i.e. receptor binding or enzyme inhibition). As differences in tolerance between healthy subjects and patients in the target population have been noted, surrogate endpoint measures could also reveal pharmacodynamic variability between these two populations. Pharmacokinetic measures can also be helpful in guiding dose selection, provided that an optimal concentration of the compound can be identified. In addition, both surrogate markers and pharmacokinetic parameters provide information on the duration of action of a compound, which can be used in the selection of dosing intervals.

Ideally, dose range and frequency should be based upon measurements of a drug's pharmacological effects over time. The dose range should ensure adequate effects at the site of action, and the dose frequency should be determined by the duration of these effects (Williams, 1992). Unfortunately, as we have discussed in the previous section, unequivocal pharmacological markers are not always available. Additionally, information on the relationship between drug concentration and effect has been difficult to ascertain for many compounds; pharmacokinetic parameters are often assessed in easily accessible fluids such as blood or urine, and differences in PK between the central compartment and peripheral measures could contribute to this difficulty.

When available, CSF levels of a central marker may be the best option to guide the selection of dose ranges and intervals at an early stage. Later studies incorporating clinical outcome measures can then be used to refine preliminary dosing strategies.

Dose-Response Relationships of CNS Compounds

There is evidence, from both surrogate endpoints and clinical outcome ratings, that the majority of CNS compounds have linear dose-response curves. In our experience with clinical trials of AD compounds, we have noted that therapeutic response is often proportional to dose (Cutler and Sramek, 1993). For example, dose-proportional inhibition of RBC cholinesterase was noted in a trial of eptastigmine in patients with AD (Sramek et al., 1995b). In a trial of physostigmine, plasma cholinesterase inhibition was linearly correlated with dose and with cognitive improvement in patients who were designated responders (Asthana et al., 1995). Dose-related improvements in verbal memory and selective reminding tests have also been observed with oral physostigmine (Beller et al., 1985; Sano et al., 1993).

The development of the AD compound, tacrine, is an example of how development can be delayed due to problems in dose selection. An early study in a small group of AD patients (n = 17) reported that beneficial effects were observed at doses up to 160 mg/day (Summers et al., 1986). These results prompted a round of larger studies which generated some controversy. For example, two studies published in 1992 reported contradictory findings on the efficacy of tacrine. In a study of 215 AD patients, Davis et al. (1992) concluded that although doses of tacrine up to 80 mg/day resulted in a significantly smaller decline in cognitive function than placebo, the difference was not large enough to be recognized by physicians in a global evaluation. Patients receiving tacrine demonstrated significantly less deterioration on the Alzheimer's Disease Assessment Scale (ADAS), but there were no differences between tacrine and placebo cohorts on the Clinical Global Impression of Change (CGIC). In contrast, another study (Farlow et al., 1992) of 468 AD patients concluded that the same dosage (80 mg/day) resulted in clinically relevant responses.

It now seems likely that the contradictory results found in these two studies were due to the deletion of higher doses of tacrine (120 and 160 mg/day) from the protocols because of a propensity to cause elevations in liver enzymes. In a large, multicenter study (n = 663), Knapp et al. (1994) found a significant dose-response relationship for tacrine at doses up to 160 mg/day. At the highest dose, significant improvement was observed on a battery of efficacy assessments, including clinician- and caregiver-rated global evaluations, quality-of-life assessments, and cognitive tests. More recent studies have confirmed the therapeutic benefit of tacrine in AD patients at higher doses (Gracon, 1996; Kaufer et al., 1996). Thus, the complications caused by tacrine's narrow therapeutic window illustrate the importance of careful dose selection to the timely completion of a drug development program.

Attempts to define dose-response relationships for antipsychotics have produced mixed results, potentially due to the diverse pharmacological profiles of these compounds. Additionally, the use of surrogate measures, such as positron emission tomography (PET), has proven difficult, as dose levels do not necessarily correspond to the level of receptor binding (Nordstrom et al., 1993; Nordstrom et al., 1995). Additionally, studies of 'classical neuroleptics' have indicated that the margin between safety and clinical efficacy is narrow. For example, in a trial of fluphenazine (n = 72), responders demonstrated the greatest improvement in positive symptoms at higher dose levels, but akathisia and EPS were also more prevalent at these doses (Levinson et al., 1995). Similarly, a controlled-dose study of haloperidol (5, 10, or 20 mg/day) in newly admitted schizophrenic patients (n = 80) indicated that 20 mg/day was superior to both the 5 and 10 mg doses on the BPRS for the first two weeks of treatment (Van Putten et al., 1990). However, by the second week, patients receiving the 20 mg dose deteriorated significantly on items such as blunted affect, motor retardation, and emotional withdrawal, potentially due to an increase in akathisia and akinesia ratings.

The advent of atypical antipsychotics fueled hopes that novel pharmacological strategies could improve the therapeutic-to-toxic index. In fact, these compounds do appear to demonstrate a superior safety profile in comparison to classical neuroleptics, increasing the probability of identifying a well-tolerated, therapeutic dose range. In a placebo-controlled, dose-ranging study of 8, 12, or 20 mg/day sertindole, dose-related improvements on the Positive and Negative Syndrome Scale (PANSS), BPRS, and CGI were observed (van Kammen et al., 1996). Although only the highest dose (20 mg) demonstrated significant superiority to placebo, this dose was very well tolerated, and the incidence of EPS was comparable to that observed in the placebo group. Clinical studies of risperidone have revealed a U-shaped dose-response curve. In a double-blind study of 135 patients with chronic schizophrenia, Chouinard et al. (1993) evaluated four doses of risperidone (2, 6, 10, and 16 mg/day) and found that all doses were indistinguishable from placebo on ratings of motor side effects. The 6 mg dose was found to be optimal, demonstrating superiority to placebo on the positive and negative subscales of the PANSS, and to haloperidol on the total PANSS and BPRS. Similarly, the Risperidone Study Group (Peuskens, 1995) evaluated the safety and efficacy of 1, 4, 8, 12, and 16 mg risperidone (n = 1362), and found that although all doses below 16 mg demonstrated superior safety to haloperidol, clinical improvement on the PANSS was optimal at doses of 4 or 8 mg. Thus, the dose-response relationships of antipsychotic compounds are clearly dependent on their individual receptor pharmacology, and require investigation early in a drug development program.

The establishment of dose-response relationships for antidepressant compounds has been particularly difficult, potentially due to delayed treatment responses or individual pharmacokinetic variability. These difficulties have led several researchers to question current dosing strategies for many antidepressant compounds. For example, Gram (1990) has suggested that inadequate dosing, coupled with the narrow therapeutic range of tricyclic antidepressants, could be responsible for the occurrence of seemingly 'drug resistant depressions.' Cain (1992) has suggested that serotonergic overstimulation due to inaccurate dosing of newer antidepressant drugs might mimic depressive symptoms, which could be mistaken for treatment failure. In his study, four patients who failed to respond to fluoxetine 20 mg/day despite apparent initial improvement underwent fluoxetine withdrawal and were restarted on a lower dose (20 mg QOD). All of these patients responded to the lower dose. Upon a retrospective analysis of the literature, Cain noted that fixed-dose studies of fluoxetine revealed increased adverse events without a corresponding increase in efficacy for doses above 5 mg/day, and decreased efficacy at doses above 40 mg/day. Cain thus concluded that current standard doses of fluoxetine may be outside the therapeutic window for some patients.

Despite these difficulties, however, several studies of various antidepressants have reported the existence of linear dose-response curves. In a multicenter, double-blind, placebo-controlled study of 50–150 mg/day fluvoxamine (n = 600), improvement on the HAM-D depressed mood item was found to be dose dependent (Walczak et al., 1996). Mendels et al. (1993) evaluated the efficacy and safety of three dose ranges of venlafaxine (25, 50–75, and 150–200 mg/day) and noted a positive dose-response trend on the HAM-D and MADRS in the first week of dosing which persisted throughout the six-week study. Linear dose-response curves have also been demonstrated for paroxetine (Tignol et al., 1992) and milnacipran (von Frenckell et al., 1990).

The variability of dose-response relationships observed with different compounds serves to illustrate the need for carefully planned dose-ranging studies in order to optimize the selection of doses for Phase II/III efficacy trials. The importance of accurate dose selection to the timely completion of a drug development program cannot be overstated.

REFERENCES

Abe K, Horiuchi M, Yoshimura K. Potentiation by DSP-4 of EEG slowing and memory impairment in basal-forebrain lesioned rats. *Eur J Pharmacol* 1997; **321**(2): 149–155.

Abelson JL, Curtis GC, Cameron OG. Hypothalamic-pituitary-adrenal axis activity in panic disorder: effects of alprazolam on 24 h secretion of adrenocorticotropin and cortisol. *J Psychiatry Res* 1996; **30**(2): 79–93.

Aguilar MT, Lemaire M, Castro P, Libotte M, Reynders J, Herchuelz A. Study of the diagnostic value of the dexamethasone suppression test in endogenous depression. *J Affect Disord* 1984; **6**(1): 33–42.

Alfredsson G, Wiesel FA. Relationships between clinical effects and monoamine metabolites and amino acids in sulpiride-treated schizophrenic patients. *Psychopharmacology (Berl)* 1990; **101**(3): 324–331.

Alhainen K, Partanen J, Reinikainen K, Lauluma V, Soininen J, Airaksinen M, Riekkinen P. Discrimination of tetrahydroaminoacridine responders by a single dose pharmaco-EEG in patients with Alzheimer's disease. *Neurosci Lett* 1991; **127**(1): 113–116.

Alvarez E, Perez-Sola V, Perez-Blanco J, Queralto JM, Torrubia R, Noguera R. Predicting outcome of lithium added to antidepressants in resistant depression. *J Affect Disord* 1997; **42**(2–3): 179–186.

Anand R, Hartman R. Strategies for the optimal development of an anti-dementia drug. Presented at the *Fifth International Conference on Alzheimer's Disease and Related Disorders*, July 24–29, 1996; Osaka, Japan.

Antuono PG. Effectiveness and safety of velnacrine for the treatment of Alzheimer's disease. A double-blind, placebo-controlled study. Mentane Study Group. *Arch Intern Med* 1995; **155**(16): 1766–1772.

Asthana S, Grieg NH, Hegedus L, Holloway HH, Raffaele KC, Shapiro MB, Soncrant TT. Clinical pharmacokinetics of physostigmine in patients with Alzheimer's disease. *Clin Pharmacol Ther* 1995; **58**(3): 299–309.

Bakish D, Cavazzoni P, Chudzik J, Ravindran A, Hrdina PD. Effects of selective serotonin reuptake inhibitors on platelet serotonin parameters in major depressive disorder. *Biol Psychiatry* 1997; **41**(2): 184–190.

Barr RD, Koekebakker M, Lawson AA, Acetylcholinesterase in the human erythron. II. Biochemical assay. *Am J Hematol* 1988; **28**: 260–265.

Barry S, Dinan TG. Neuroendocrine challenge tests in depression: a study of growth hormone, TRH, and cortisol release. *J Affect Disord* 1990; **18**(4): 229–234.

Beasley CM Jr, Sanger T, Satterlee W, Tollefson G, Tran P, Hamilton S. Olanzapine versus placebo: results of a double-blind, fixed-dose olanzapine trial. *Psychopharmacology (Berl)* 1996; **124**(1–2): 159–167.

Beller SA, Overall JE, Swann AC. Efficacy of oral physostigmine in primary degenerative dementia. A double-blind study of response to different dose levels. *Psychopharmacology (Berl)* 1985; **87**(2): 147–151.

Bertilsson L, Tuck JR, Siwers B. Biochemical effects of zimelidine in man. *Eur J Clin Pharmacol* 1980; **18**(6): 483–487.

Biegon A, Essar N, Isreaeli M, Elizur A, Bruch S, Bar-Nathan AA. Serotonin 5-HT2 receptor binding on blood platelets as a state dependent marker in major affective disorder. *Psychopharmacology (Berl)* 1990b; **102**(1): 73–75.

Biegon A, Grinspoon A, Blumenfeld B, Bleich A, Apter A, Mester R. Increased serotonin 5-HT$_2$ receptor binding on blood platelets of suicidal men. *Psychopharmacology (Berl)* 1990a; **100**(2): 165–176.

Bjorklund M, Jakala P, Schmidt B, Riekkinen M, Koivisto E, Riekkinen P Jr. An indirect cholinesterase inhibitor, metrifonate, increases neocortical EEG arousal in rats. *Neuroreport* 1996; **7**(5): 1097–1101.

Bowers MB, Swigar ME, Jatlow PI, Goicoechea N. Plasma catecholamine metabolism and early response to haloperidol. *J Clin Psychiatry* 1984; **45**: 284–291.

Bowers MB, Swigar ME, Jatlow PI, Hoffman FJ, Goicoechea N. Correlates of early neuroleptic response using a uniform haloperidol dose. *Int Clin Psychopharmacol* 1987; **2**(3): 255–260.

Buysse DJ, Reynolds CF 3rd, Hoch CC, Houck PR, Kupfer DJ, Mazumdar S, Frank E. Longitudinal effects of nortriptyline on EEG sleep and the likelihood of recurrence in elderly depressed patients. *Neuropsychopharmacology* 1996; **14**(4): 243–252.

Cain JW. Poor response to fluoxetine: underlying depression, serotonergic overstimulation, or a 'therapeutic window'? *J Clin Psychiatry* 1992; **53**(8): 272–277.

Calloway SP, Dolan RJ, Fonagy P, DeSouza VF, Wakeling A. Endocrine changes and clinical profiles in depression: I. The dexamethasone suppression test. *Psychol Med* 1984; **14**(4): 749–758.

Canal N, Imbimbo BP. Relationship between pharmacodynamic activity and cognitive effects of eptastigmine in patients with Alzheimer's disease. Eptastigmine Study Group. *Clin Pharmacol Ther* 1996; **60**(2): 218–228.

Carroll BJ, Curtis GC, Davies BM, Mendels J, Sugarman AA. Urinary free cortisol excretion in depression. *Psychol Med* 1976b; **6**: 43–60.

Carroll BJ, Curtis GC, Mendels J. Neuroendocrine regulation in depression. II. Discrimination of depressed from nondepressed patients. *Arch Gen Psychiatry* 1976a; **33**(9): 1051–1058.

Carroll BJ, Feinberg M, Greden JF, Tarika J, Albala AA, Haskett RF, James NM, Kronfol Z, Lohr N, Steiner M, de Vigne JP, Young E. A specific laboratory test for the diagnosis of melancholia. Standardization, validation, and clinical utility. *Arch Gen Psychiatry* 1981; **38**(1): 15–22.

Celada P, Perez J, Alvarez E, Artigas F. Monoamine oxidase inhibitors phenelzine and brofaromine increase plasma serotonin and decrease 5-hydroxyindolacetic acid in patients with major depression: relationship to clinical improvement. *J Clin Psychopharmacol* 1992; **12**(5): 305–315.

Chang JP, Yu KL, Wong AO, Peter RE. Differential actions of dopamine receptor subtypes on gonadotropin and growth hormone release in vitro in goldfish. *Neuroendocrinology* 1990; **51**(6): 664–674.

Chouinard G, Jones B, Remington G, Bloom D, Addington D, MacEwan GW, Labelle A, Beauclair L, Arnott W. A Canadian multicenter placebo-controlled study of fixed doses of risperidone and haloperidol in the treatment of chronic schizophrenic patients. *J Clin Psychopharmacol* 1993; **13**(1): 25–40.

Cleare AJ, Murray RM, O'Keane V. Reduced prolactin and cortisol responses to d-fenfluramine in depressed compared to healthy matched control subjects. *Neuropsychopharmacology* 1996; **14**(5): 349–354.

Cowen PJ, Anderson IM, Grahame-Smith DG. Neuroendocrine effects of azapirones. *J Clin Psychopharmacol* 1990; **10**(3 Suppl): 21–25.

Curtis VA, Wright P, Reveley A, Kerwin R, Lucey JV. Effect of clozapine on d-fenfluramine-evoked neuroendocrine responses in schizophrenia and its relationship to clinical improvement. *Br J Psychiatry* 1995; **166**(5): 642–646.

Cutler NR, Haxby J, Kay AD, Narang PK, Lesko LJ, et al. Evaluation of zimeldine in Alzheimer's disease: cognitive and biochemical measures. *Arch Neurol* 1985; **42**: 744–748.

Cutler NR, Sramek JJ. Proper development for Alzheimer's disease [letter]. *N Engl J Med* 1993; **328**: 808.

Cutler NR, Sramek JJ. Scientific and ethical concerns in clinical trials in Alzheimer's patients: the bridging study. *Eur J Clin Pharmacol* 1995a; **48**: 421–428.

Cutler NR, Sramek JJ. The target population in phase I clinical trials of cholinergic compounds in Alzheimer's disease: the role of the 'bridging study.' *Alzheimer Dis Assoc Disorders* 1995b; **9**:139–145.

Cutler NR, Sramek JJ, Kilborn JR. The bridging concept: optimizing the dose for phase II/III in Alzheimer's disease. *Neurodegeneration* 1996; **5**(4): 511–514.

Cutler NR, Sramek JJ, Veroff AE. *Alzheimer's Disease: Optimizing Drug Development Strategies*. Chichester: John Wiley & Sons, 1994.

Davidson M, Kahn RS, Stern RG, Hirschowitz J, Apter S, Knott P, Davis KL. Treatment with clozapine and its effect on plasma homovanillic acid and norepinephrine concentrations in schizophrenia. *Psychiatry Res* 1993; **46**(2): 151–163.

Davila R, Manero E, Zumarraga M, Andia I, et al. Plasma homovanillic acid as a predictor of response to neuroleptics. *Arch Gen Psychiatry* 1988; **45**(6): 564–567.

Davis KL, Thal LJ, Gamzu ER, Davis CS, Woolson RF, Gracon SI, Drachman DA, Schneider LS, Whitehouse PJ, Hoover TM, et al. A double-blind, placebo-controlled, multicenter study of tacrine for Alzheimer's disease. *N Engl J Med* 1992; **327**: 1253–1259.

DeBellis MD, Geracioti TD Jr, Altelmus M, Kling MA. Cerebrospinal fluid monoamine metabolites in fluoxetine-treated patients with major depression and in healthy volunteers. *Biol Psychiatry* 1993; **33**(8–9): 636–641.

Delgado PL, Price LH, Miller HL, Salomon RM, Licinio J, Krystal JH, Heninger GR, Charney DS. Rapid serotonin depletion as a provocative challenge test for patients with major depression: relevance to antidepressant action and the neurobiology of depression. *Psychopharmacol Bull* 1991; **27**(3): 321–330.

Duncan E, Wolkin A, Angrist B, Sanfilipo M, Wieland S, Cooper TB, Rotrosen J. Plasma homovanillic acid in neuroleptic responsive and nonresponsive schizophrenics. *Biol Psychiatry* 1993; **34**(8): 523–528.

Ellman GL, Courtney KD, Andres V, Featherstone RM. A new and rapid colorimetric determination of acetylcholinesterase activity. *Biochem Pharmacol* 1961; **7**: 88–95.

Elmstahl S, Rosen I, Gullberg B. Quantitative EEG in elderly patients with Alzheimer's disease and healthy controls. *Dementia* 1994; **5**(2): 119–124.

Extein I, Pottash AL, Gold MS. Number of cortisol time-points and dexamethasone suppression test sensitivity for major depression. *Psychoneuroendocrinology* 1985; **10**(3): 281–288.

Faraone SV, Brown WA, Laughren TP. Serum neuroleptic levels, prolactin levels, and relapse: a two-year study of schizophrenic outpatients. *J Clin Psychiatry* 1987; **48**(4): 151–154.

Faraone SV, Curran JP, Laughren T, Faltus F, Johnston R, Brown WA. Neuroleptic bioavailability, psychosocial factors, and clinical status: a 1-year study of schizophrenic outpatients after dose reduction. *Psychiatry Res* 1986; **19**(4): 311–322.

Farlow M, Gracon SI, Hershey LA, et al. A controlled trial of tacrine in Alzheimer's disease. *JAMA* 1992; **268**: 2523–2529.

Fleming TR, DeMets DL. Surrogate end points in clinical trials: are we being misled? *Ann Intern Med* 1996; **125**: 605–613.

Fontaine R, Ontiveros A, Elie R, Kensler TT, Roberts DL, Kaplita S, Ecker JA, Faludi G. A double-blind comparison of nefazodone, imipramine, and placebo in major depression. *J Clin Psychiatry* 1994; **55**(6): 234–241.

Garcia A, Galinowski A, Guicheney P, Mignot E, et al. Free and conjugated plasma homovanillic acid in schizophrenic patients. *Biol Psychiatry* 1989; **26**(1): 87–96.

Gibbons RD, Hedeker D, Davis JM. Regression toward the mean: more on the price of beer and the salaries of priests. *Psychoneuroendocrinology* 1987; **12**(3): 185–192.

Goodwin FK, Post RM. Catecholamine metabolite studies in the affective disorders: issues of specificity and significance. In: Usdin E, Hamburg DA, Barchas JD (eds.) *Neuroregulators and Psychiatric Disorders*. New York: Oxford University Press, Inc., 1977, p. 135–145.

Gracon SI. Evaluation of tacrine hydrochloride (Cognex) in two parallel-group studies. *Acta Neurol Scand Suppl* 1996; **165**: 114–122.

Grahame-Smith DG. Serotonin function in affective disorders. *Acta Psychiatr Scand Suppl* 1989; **350**: 7–12.

Gram LF. Inadequate dosing and pharmacokinetic variability as confounding factors in assessment of efficacy of antidepressants. *Clin Neuropharmacol* 1990; **13**(Suppl 1): 35–44.

Green AI, Alam MY, Sobieraj JT, Pappalardo KM, Waternauz C, Salzman C, Schatzberg AF, Schildkraut JJ, Clozapine response and plasma catecholamines and their metabolites. *Psychiatry Res* 1993; **46**(2): 139–149.

Groenink L, Van der Gugten J, Verdouw PM, Maes RA, Olivier B. The anxiolytic effects of flesinoxan, a 5-HT1A receptor agonist, are not related to its neuroendocrine effects. *Eur J Pharmacol* 1995; **280**(2): 185–193.

Gustafson L. Physostigmine and tetrahydroaminoacridine treatment of Alzheimer's disease. *Acta Neurol Scand Suppl* 1993; **149**(Rand): 39–41.

Hallack M, Giacobini E. A comparison of the effects of two inhibitors on brain cholinesterase. *Neuropharmacology* 1987; **28**: 199–206.

Hallack M, Giacobini E. Physostigmine, tacrine, and metrifonate: the effect of multiple dosage on acetylcholine in rat brain. *Neuropharmacology* 1989; **28**: 199–206.

Heuser IJ, Schweiger U, Gotthardt U, Schmider J, Lammers CH, Dettling M, Yassouridis A, Holsboer F. Pituitary-adrenal system regulation and psychopathology during amitriptyline treatment in elderly depressed patients and normal comparison subjects. *Am J Psychiatry* 1996; **153**(1): 93–99.

Hirschowitz J, Hitzemann R, Piscani K, Burr G, Frecska E, Culliton D, Mann M, Curtis C. The Dose Reduction in Schizophrenia (DORIS) Study: a final report. *Schizophr Res* 1997; **23**(1): 31–43.

Hrdina PD, Bakish D, Chudzik J, Ravindran A, Lapierre YD. Serotonergic markers in platelets of patients with major depression: upregulation of 5-HT2 receptors. *J Psychiatry Neurosci* 1995; **20**(1): 11–19.

Hsiao JK, Agren H, Bartko JJ, Rodorfer MV, Linnoila M, Potter WZ. Monoamine neurotransmitter interactions and the prediction of antidepressant response. *Arch Gen Psychiatry* 1987; **44**(12): 1078–1083.

Hubain PP, Castro P, Mesters P, De Maertelaer V, Mendlewicz J. Alprazolam and amitriptyline in the treatment of major depressive disorder: a double-blind clinical and sleep EEG study. *J Affect Disord* 1990; **18**(1): 67–73.

Hubain PP, Souery D, Jonck L, Staner L, Van Veeren C, Kerkhofs M, Mendlewicz
    J, Linkowski P. Relationship between the Newcastle scale and sleep
    polysomnographic variables in major depression: a controlled study. *Eur
    Neuropsychopharmacol* 1995; **5**(2): 129–134.
Katz MM, Maas J, Frazer A, Koslow SH, Bowden CL, Berman N, Swann AC,
    Stokes PE. Drug-induced actions on brain neurotransmitter systems and
    changes   in   the   behaviors   and   emotions   of   depressed   patients.
    Neuropsychopharmacology 1994; **11**(2): 89–100.
Kaufer DI, Cummings JL, Christine D. Effect of tacrine on behavioral symptoms in
    Alzheimer's disease: an open-label study. *J Geriatr Psychiatry Neurol* 1996;
    9(1): 1–6.
Kendler KS, Heniger GR, Roth RH. Brain contribution to the haloperidol-induced
    increase in plasma homovanillic acid. *Eur J Pharmacol* 1981; **71**(2–3): 321–
    326.
Knapp MJ, Knopman DS, Solomon PR, Pendlebury WW, Davis CS, Gracon SI. A
    30-week randomized controlled trial of high-dose tacrine in patients with
    Alzheimer's disease. The Tacrine Study Group. *JAMA* 1994; **271**(13): 985–
    991.
Konicki PE, Owen RR, Litman RE, Pickar D. The acute effects of central- and
    peripheral-acting dopamine antagonists on plasma HVA in schizophrenic
    patients. *Life Sci* 1991; **48**(14): 1411–1416.
Lawson AA, Barr RD. Acetylcholinesterase in red blood cells. *Am J Hematol*
    1987; **26**: 101–112.
Lee HS, Kim CH, Song DH, Choi NK, Yoo KJ. Clozapine does not elevate serum
    prolactin levels in healthy men. *Biol Psychiatry* 1995; **38**(11): 762–764.
Leonard BE. Serotonin receptors and their function in sleep, anxiety disorders and
    depression. *Psychother Psychosom* 1996; **65**(2): 66–75.
Lerer B, Gillon D, Lichtenberg P, Gorgine M, Gelfin Y, Shapira B.
    Interrelationship of age, depression, and central serotonergic function:
    evidence from fenfluramine challenge studies. *Int Psychogeriatr* 1996; **8**(1):
    83–102.
Lesch KP, Wiesmann M, Hoh A, Muller T, Disselkamp-Tietze J, Osterheider M,
    Schulte HM. 5-HT1A receptor-effector system responsivity in panic disorder.
    Psychopharmacology (Berl) 1992; **106**(1): 111–117.
Levinson DF, Simpson GM, Lo ES, Cooper TB, Singh H, Yadalam K, Stephanos
    MJ. Fluphenazine plasma levels, dosage, efficacy, and side effects. *Am J
    Psychiatry* 1995; **152**(5): 765–771.
Levy AD, Van de Kar LD. Endocrine and receptor pharmacology of serotonergic
    anxiolytics, antipsychotics, and antidepressants. *Life Sci* 1992; **51**(2): 83–94.
Lichtenberg P, Shapira B, Gillon D, Kindler S, Cooper TB, Newman ME, Lerer B.
    Hormone responses to fenfluramine and placebo challenge in endogenous
    depression. *Psychiatry Res* 1992; **43**(2): 137–146.

Lieberman JA, Kane JM, Safferman AZ, Pollack S, Howard A, Szymanski S, Masiar SJ, Kronig MH, Cooper T, Novacenko H. Predictors of response to clozapine. *J Clin Psychiatry* 1994; **55**(Suppl B): 126–128.

Lindstrom LH. Low HVA and normal 5-HIAA CSF levels in drug-free schizophrenic patients compared to healthy volunteers: correlations to symptomatology and family history. *Psychiatry Res* 1985; **14**(4): 265–273.

Lopez AL, Kathol RG, Noyes R Jr. Reduction in urinary free cortisol during benzodiazepine treatment of panic disorder. *Psychoneuroendocrinology* 1990; **15**(1): 23–28.

Lopez OL, Brenner RP, Becker JT, Ulrich RF, Boller F, DeKosky ST. EEG spectral abnormalities and psychosis as predictors of cognitive and functional decline in probable Alzheimer's disease. *Neurology* 1997; **48**(6): 1521–1525.

Malone KM, Corbitt EM, Li S, Mann JJ. Prolactin response to fenfluramine and suicide attempt lethality in major depression. *Br J Psychiatry* 1996; **168**(3): 324–329.

Mamelok R. How controversial are surrogate endpoints? *Biotechnology* 1994; **12**: 134–135.

Mann JJ, McBride PA, Malone KM, DeMeo M, Keilp J. Blunted serotonergic responsivity in depressed inpatients. *Neuropsychopharmacology* 1995; **13**(1): 53–64.

Markianos M, Alevizos B, Hatzimanolis J, Stefanis C. Effects of monoamine oxidase A inhibition on plasma biogenic amine metabolites in depressed patients. *Psychiatry Res* 1994; **52**(3): 259–264.

Martensson B, Wagner A, Beck O, Brodin K, Montero D, Asberg M. Effects of clomipramine treatment on cerebrospinal fluid monoamine metabolites and platelet 3H-imipramine binding and serotonin uptake and concentration in major depressive disorder. *Acta Psychiatr Scand* 1991; **83**(2): 125–133.

Mazure CM, Nelson JC, Jatlow PI, Bowers MB. Plasma free homovanillic acid (HVA) as a predictor of clinical response in acute psychosis. *Biol Psychiatry* 1991; **30**(5): 475–482.

Megens AA, Awouters FH, Schotte A, Meert TF, Dugovic C, Niemegeers CJ, Leysen JE. Survey on the pharmacodynamics of the new antipsychotic risperidone. *Psychopharmacology (Berl)* 1994; **114**(1): 9–23.

Meltzer HY, Busch D. Serum prolactin response to chlorpromazine and psychopathology in schizophrenics: implications for the dopamine hypothesis. *Psychiatry Res* 1983; **9**(4): 285–299.

Meltzer HY, Busch DA, Fang VS. Serum neuroleptic and prolactin levels in schizophrenic patients and clinical response. *Psychiatry Res* 1983; **9**(4): 271–283.

Mendels J, Johnston R, Mattes J, Reisenberg R. Efficacy and safety of b.i.d. doses of venlafaxine in a dose-response study. *Psychopharmacol Bull* 1993; **29**(2): 169–174.

Mendlewicz J, Kerkhofs M. Sleep electroencephalography in depressive illness. A collaborative study by the World Health Organization. *Br J Psychiatry* 1991; **159**: 505–509.

Minthon L, Gustafson L, Dalfelt G, Hagberg B, Nilsson K, Risberg J, Rosen I, Seiving B, Wendt PE. Oral tetrahydroaminoacridine treatment of Alzheimer's disease evaluated clinically and by regional cerebral blood flow and EEG. *Dementia* 1993; **4**(1): 32–42.

Mitchell P, Smythe G. Hormonal responses to fenfluramine in depressed and control subjects. *J Affect Disord* 1990; **19**(1): 43–51.

Muller-Spahn F, Ackenheil M, Albus M, May G, Naber D, Welter D, Zander K. Neuroendocrine effects of apomorphine in chronic schizophrenic patients under long-term neuroleptic therapy and after drug withdrawal: relations to psychopathology and tardive dyskinesia. *Psychopharmacology (Berl)* 1984; **84**(3): 436–440.

Nagaoka S, Iwamoto N, Arai H. First-episode neuroleptic-free schizophrenics: concentrations of monoamines and their metabolites in plasma and their correlations with clinical responses to haloperidol treatment. *Biol Psychiatry* 1997; **41**(8): 857–864.

Newman LM, Johnson EM, Staples RE. Assessment of the effectiveness of animal developmental toxicity testing for human safety. *Reprod Toxicol* 1993; **7**(4): 359–390.

Nofzinger EA, Reynolds CF, Thase ME, Frank E, Jennings JR, Fasiczka AL, Sullivan LR, Kupfer DJ. REM sleep enhancement by bupropion in depressed men. *Am J Psychiatry* 1995; **152**(2): 274–276.

Nordstrom AL, Farde L, Halldin C. High 5-HT2 receptor occupancy in clozapine treated patients demonstrated by PET. *Psychopharmacology* 1993; **110**(3): 365–367.

Nordstrom AL, Farde L, Nyberg S, Karlsson P, et al. D1, D2, and 5-HT2 receptor occupancy in relation to clozapine serum concentration: a PET study of schizophrenic patients. *Am J Psychiatry* 1995; **152**(10): 1444–1449.

Norman TR, Apostolopoulos M, Burrows GD, Judd FK. Neuroendocrine responses to single doses of buspirone in obsessive compulsive disorder. *Int Clin Psychopharmacol* 1994; **9**(2): 89–94.

O'Keane V, Dinan TG. Prolactin and cortisol responses to d-fenfluramine in major depression: evidence for diminished responsivity of central serotonergic function. *Am J Psychiatry* 1991; **148**(8): 1009–1015.

O'Keane V, McLoughlin D, Dinan TG. D-fenfluramine-induced prolactin and cortisol release in major depression: response to treatment. *J Affect Disord* 1992; **26**(3): 143–150.

Ortiz J, Mariscor C, Alvarez E, Artigas F. Effects of the antidepressant drug tianeptine on plasma and platelet serotonin of depressive patients and healthy controls. *J Affect Disord* 1993; **29**(4): 227–234.

Pandey GN, Pandey SC, Dwivedi Y, Sharma RP, Janicak PG, Davis JM. Platelet serotonin-2A receptors: a potential biological marker for suicidal behavior. *Am J Psychiatry* 1995; **152**(6): 850–855.

Pandurangi AK, Narasimhachari N, Blackard WG, Landa BS. Relation of serum molindone levels to serum prolactin levels and antipsychotic response. *J Clin Psychiatry* 1989; **50**(10): 379–381.

Passero S, Rocchi R, Vatti G, Burgalassi L, Battistini N. Quantitative EEG mapping, regional cerebral blood flow, and neuropsychological function in Alzheimer's disease. *Dementia* 1995; **6**(3): 148–156.

Perryman KM, Fitten LJ. Quantitative EEG during a double-blind trial of THA and lecithin in patients with Alzheimer's disease. *J Geriatr Psychiatry Neurol* 1991; **4**(3): 127–133.

Peselow ED, Baxter N, Fieve RR, Barouche F. The dexamethasone suppression test as a monitor of clinical recovery. *Am J Psychiatry* 1987; **144**(1): 30–35.

Peselow ED, Goldring N, Fieve RR, Wright R. The dexamethasone suppression test in depressed outpatients and normal control subjects. *Am J Psychiatry* 1983; **140**(2): 245–247.

Peuskens J. Risperidone in the treatment of patients with chronic schizophrenia: a multi-national, mutli-centre, double-blind, parallel-group study versus haloperidol. Risperidone Study Group. *Br J Psychiatry* 1995; **166**(6): 712–726.

Pickar D, Breier A, Kelsoe J. Plasma homovanillic acid as an index of central dopaminergic activity: studies in schizophrenic patients. *Ann NY Acad Sci* 1988; **537**: 339–346.

Pickar D, Labarca R, Doran AR, Wolkowitz OM, et al. Longitudinal measurement of plasma homovanillic acid levels in schizophrenic patients. Correlation with psychosis and response to neuroleptic treatment. *Arch Gen Psychiatry* 1986; **43**(7): 669–676.

Poland RE, Rubin RT, Lesser IM, Lane LA, Hart PJ. Neuroendocrine aspects of primary endogenous depression: serum dexamethasone concentrations and hypothalamic-pituitary-adrenal cortical activity as determinants of the dexamethasone suppression test response. *Arch Gen Psychiatry* 1987; **44**: 790–795.

Polinsky RJ, Homes KV, Brown RT, Weise V. CSF acetylcholinesterase levels are reduced in multiple system atrophy with autonomic failure. *Neurology* 1989; **39**: 40–44.

Potter WZ, Scheinin M, Golden RN, Rudorfer MV, Cowdry RW, Calil HM, Ross RJ, Linnoila M. Selective antidepressants and cerebrospinal fluid. Lack of specificity on norepinephrine and serotonin metabolites. *Arch Gen Psychiatry* 1985; **42**(12): 1171–1177.

Prentice RL. Surrogate endpoints in clinical trials: definition and operational criteria. *Stat Med* 1989; **8**: 431–440.

Prichep LS, John ER, Ferris SH, Reisberg B, Almas M, Alper K, Cancro R. Quantitative EEG correlates of cognitive deterioration in the elderly. *Neurobiol Aging* 1994; **15**(1): 85–90.

Primavera A, Novello P, Finocchi C, Canevari E, Corsello L. Correlation between mini-mental state examination and quantitative electroencephalography in senile dementia of Alzheimer type. *Neuropsychobiology* 1990; **23**(2): 74–78.

Quintana J. Platelet serotonin and plasma tryptophan decreases in endogenous depression. Clinical, therapeutic, and biological correlations. *J Affect Disord* 1992; **24**(2): 55–62.

Radat F, Morand P. Prediction of therapeutic response in depressive states. *Ann Med Psychol (Paris) 1996*; **154**(2): 89–102.

Ribeiro SC, Tandon R, Grunhaus L, Greden JF. The DST as a predictor of outcome in depression: a meta-analysis. *Am J Psychiatry* 1993; **150**(11): 1618–1629.

Rickels K, Robinson DS, Schweizer E, Marcus RN, Roberts DL. Nefazodone: aspects of efficacy. *J Clin Psychiatry* 1995; **56**(Suppl 6): 43–46.

Rogers SL, Friedhoff LT. The efficacy and safety of donepezil in patients with Alzheimer's disease: results of a US multicentre, randomized, double-blind, placebo-controlled trial. The Donepezil Study Group. *Dementia* 1996; **7**(6): 293–303.

Roy-Byrne PP, Cowley DS, Hommer D, Ritchie J, Greenblatt D, Nemeroff C. Neuroendocrine effects of diazepam in panic and generalized anxiety disorders. *Biol Psychiatry* 1991; **30**(1): 73–80.

Rubin RT, Poland RE, Lesser IM, Winston RA, Blodgett NAL. Neuroendocrine aspects of primary endogenous depression: cortisol secretory dynamics in patients and matched controls. *Arch Gen Psychiatry* 1987; **44**: 328–226.

Rush AJ, Weissenburger J, Vasavada N, Orsulak PJ, Fairchild CJ. Dexamethasone suppression test status does not predict differential response to nortriptyline versus amitriptyline. *J Clin Psychopharmacol* 1988; **8**(6): 421–425.

Sano M, Bell K, Marder K, Stricks L, Stern Y, Mayeux R. Safety and efficacy of oral physostigmine in the treatment of Alzheimer's disease. *Clin Neuropharmacol* 1993; **16**(1): 61–69.

Sanz P, Rodriquez-Vicente MC, Diaz D, et al. Red blood cell and total blood cell acetylcholinesterase and plasma pseudocholinesterase in humans: observed variances. *Clin Toxicol* 1991; **29**: 81–90.

Scatton B, Zarifian E, Bianchetti G, Cuche H, et al. Use of haloperidol in high doses in schizophrenia: clinical, biochemical, and pharmacokinetic study. *Encephale* 1982; **8**(1): 1–8.

Scheinin M, Syvalahti EK, Hietala J, Huupponen R, Pihlajamaki K, Seppala OP, Sako E. Effects of apomorphine on blood levels of homovanillic acid, growth hormone and prolactin in medicated schizophrenics and healthy control subjects. *Prog Neuropsychopharmacol Biol Psychiatry* 1985; **9**(4): 441–449.

Schlegel S, Schlosser R, Hiemke C, Nickel O, Bockisch A, Hahn K. Prolactin plasma levels and D2-dopamine receptor occupancy measured with IBZM-SPECT. *Psychopharmacology (Berl)* 1996; **124**(3): 285–287.

Schreiter-Gasser U, Gasser T, Ziegler P. Quantitative EEG analysis in early onset Alzheimer's disease: correlations with severity, clinical characteristics, visual EEG, and CCT. *Electroencephalograph Clin Neurophysiol* 1994; **90**(4): 267–272.

Seiler W, Wetzel H, Hillert A, Schollnhammer G, Benkert O, Hiemke C. Plasma levels of benperidol, prolactin, and homovanillic acid after intravenous versus two different kinds of oral application of the neuroleptic in schizophrenic patients. *Exp Clin Endocrinol* 1994; **102**(4): 326–333.

Shannon HE, Bymaster FP, Calligaro DO, Greenwood B, Mitch CH, Sawyer BD, Ward JS, Wong DT, Olesen PH, Sheardown MJ, et al. Xanomeline: a novel muscarinic receptor agonist with functional selectivity for M1 receptors. *J Pharmacol Exp Ther* 1994; **269**(1): 271–281.

Sharpley AL, Walsh AE, Cowen PJ. Nefazodone—a novel antidepressant—may increase REM sleep. *Biol Psychiatry* 1992; **31**: 1070–1073.

Sheline Y, Bardgett ME, Csernansky JG. Correlated reductions in cerebrospinal fluid 5-HIAA and MHPG concentrations after treatment with selective serotonin reuptake inhibitors. *J Clin Psychopharmacol* 1997; **17**(1): 11–14.

Sheline YI, Bardgett ME, Jackson JL, Newcomer JW, Csernansky JG. Platelet serotonin markers and depressive symptomatology. *Biol Psychiatry* 1995; **37**(7): 442–447.

Shigeta M, Persson A, Viitanen M, Winblad B, Nordberg A. EEG regional changes during long-term treatment with tetrahydroaminoacridine (THA) in Alzheimer's disease. *Acta Neurol Scand Suppl* 1993; **149**: 58–61.

Sirviö J, Kutvonen R, Koininen H, Hartikainen P, Riekkinen PJ. Cholinesterases in the cerebrospinal fluid, plasma, and erythrocytes of patients with Alzheimer's disease. *J Neural Transm* 1989; **75**: 119–127.

Sonntag A, Rothe B, Guldner J, Yassouridis A, Holsboer F, Steiger A. Trimipramine and imipramine exert different effects on the sleep EEG and on nocturnal hormone secretion during treatment of major depression. *Depression* 1996; **4**(1): 1–13.

Spreux-Varoquaux O, Gailledreau J, Vanier B, Bothua D, Plas J, Chevalier JF, Advenier C, Pays M, Brion S. Initial increase of plasma serotonin: a biological predictor for the antidepressant response to clomipramine? *Biol Psychiatry* 1996; **40**(6): 465–473.

Sramek JJ, Block GA, Reines SA, Sawin SF, Barchowsky A, Cutler NR. A multiple-dose safety trial of eptastigmine in Alzheimer's disease, with pharmacodynamic observations of red blood cell cholinesterase. *Life Sci* 1995b; **56**(5): 319–326.

Sramek JJ, Cutler NR, Hurley DJ, Seifert RD. The utility of salivary amylase as an evaluation of M3 muscarinic agonist activity in Alzheimer's disease. *Prog Neuropsychopharmacol Biol Psychiatry* 1995a; **19**(1): 85–91.

Stahl SM, Hauger RL, Rausch JL, Fleishaker JC, Hubbell-Alberts E. Downregulation of serotonin receptor subtypes by nortriptyline and adinazolam in major depressive disorder: neuroendocrine and platelet markers. *Clin Neuropharmacol* 1993; **16**(Suppl 3): S19–S31.

Staner L, Kerkhofs M, Detroux D, Leyman S, Linkowski P, Mendlewicz J. Acute, subchronic and withdrawal sleep EEG changes during treatment with paroxetine and amitriptyline: a double-blind, randomized trial in major depression. *Sleep* 1995; **18**(6): 470–477.

St. Clair DM, Brock DJH, Barron L. A monoclonal antibody technique for plasma and red cell acetylcholinesterase activity in Alzheimer's disease. *J Neurol Sci* 1986; **73**: 169–176.

Stefanis CN, Alevizos B, Markianos M, Hatzimanolis J. Effect of moclobemide on clinical and neurochemical variables in depressed patients (preliminary findings). *J Neural Transm Suppl* 1988; **26**: 87–95.

Stokes PE, Stoll PL, Koslow SH, Maas JW, Davis JM, Swann AC, Robins E. Pretreatment DST and hypothalamic-pituitary-adrenocortical function in depressed patients and comparison groups. *Arch Gen Psychiatry* 1984; **41**(3): 257–267.

Summers W, Majoski L, Marik G, Tachiki K, Kling A. Oral tetrahydroaminoacridine in long-term treatment of senile dementia, Alzheimer type. *N Engl J Med* 1986; **315**: 1241–1245.

Thase ME, Kupfer DJ, Buysse DJ, Frank E, Simons AD, McEachran AB, Rashid KF, Grochocinski VJ. Electroencephalographic sleep profiles in single-episode and recurrent forms of major depression: I. Comparison during acute depressive states. *Biol Psychiatry* 1995; **38**(8): 506–515.

Thomsen T, Kaden B, Fisher JP, et al. Inhibition of acetylcholinesterase activity in human brain tissue and erythrocytes by galanthamine, physostigmine, and tacrine. *Eur J Clin Chem Clin Biochem* 1991; **29**: 487–492.

Tignol J, Stoker MJ, Dunbar GC. Paroxetine in the treatment of melancholia and severe depression. *Int Clin Psychopharmacol* 1992; **7**(2): 91–94.

Twardowska K, Rybakowski J. Limbic-hypothalamic-pituitary-adrenal axis in depression: literature review. *Psychiatr Pol* 1996; **30**(5): 741–755.

van Bemmel AL, Havermans RG, van Diest R. Effects of trazodone on EEG sleep and clinical state in major depression. *Psychopharmacology (Berl)* 1992; **107**(4): 569–574.

van Kammen DP, McEvoy JP, Targum SD, Kardatzke D, Sebree TB. A randomized, controlled, dose-ranging trial of sertindole in patients with schizophrenia. *Psychopharmacology (Berl)* 1996; **124**(1–2): 168–175.

Van Putten T, Marder SR, Mintz J. A controlled dose comparison of haloperidol in newly admitted schizophrenic patients. *Arch Gen Psychiatry* 1990; **47**(8): 754–758.

von Frenckell R, Ansseau M, Serre C, Sutet P. Pooling two controlled comparisons of milnacipran (F2207) and amitriptyline in endogenous inpatients. A new approach in dose ranging studies. *Int Clin Psychopharmacol* 1990; **5**(1): 49–56.

Walczak DD, Apter JT, Halikas JA, Borison RL, Carman JS, Post GL, Patrick R, Cohn JB, Cunningham LA, Rittbreg B, Preskorn SH, Kang JS, Wilcox CS. The oral dose-effect relationship for fluvoxamine: a fixed-dose comparison against placebo in depressed outpatients. *Ann Clin Psychiatry* 1996; **8**(3): 139–151.

Wetzel H, Szegedi A, Hain C, Wiesner J, Schlegel S, Benkert O. Seroquel (ICI 204 636), a putative 'atypical' antipsychotic, in schizophrenia with positive symptomatology: results of an open clinical trial and changes of neuroendocrinological and EEG parameters. *Psychopharmacology (Berl)* 1995; **119**(2): 231–238.

Wiedemann K, Kellner M. Endocrine characterization of the new dopamine autoreceptor agonist roxindole. *Exp Clin Endocrinol* 1994; **102**(4): 284–288.

Williams RL. Dosage regimen design: pharmacodynamic considerations. *J Clin Pharmacol* 1992; **32**: 597–602.

Wong AO, Chang JP, Peter RE. In vitro and in vivo evidence that dopamine exerts growth hormone-releasing activity in goldfish. *Am J Physiol* 1993; **264**(6): 925–932.

Zemlan FP, Garver DL. Depression and antidepressant therapy: receptor dynamics. *Prog Neuropsychopharmacol Biol Psychiatry* 1990; **14**(4): 503–523.

Zemlan FP, Hirschowitz J, Sautter F, Garver DL. Relationship of psychotic symptom clusters in schizophrenia to neuroleptic treatment and growth hormone response to apomorphine. *Psychiatry Res* 1986; **18**(3): 239–255.

4   Design options

The design of a clinical trial is based on several factors, including the particular question under investigation, regulatory requirements, practical concerns, and ethical issues. Additionally, there are some considerations that are specific to particular types of CNS compounds or indications.

STUDY DURATION

Many CNS compounds require a substantial amount of time before their beneficial effects can be detected. In outpatient trials of antidepressants, a period of 4–6 weeks is often necessary before clear distinctions between placebo and active drug can be discerned (Quitkin et al., 1984). Indeed, in a placebo-controlled study of ABT-200 and fluoxetine, a treatment period of eight weeks was necessary to detect an effect (Sramek et al., 1994/1995). However, Klein (1991) has noted that many antidepressant trials employ a treatment period of only three weeks, which makes the detection of efficacy unlikely. In this situation, various nonspecific drug effects, such as sedation, could be mistaken for true therapeutic benefit.

In anxiolytic trials, the double-blind, randomized treatment period should also last at least four weeks. Four weeks became the standard for anxiolytic trials with the development of the benzodiazepines, as patients generally demonstrate some improvement within 1–2 weeks (Cutler et al., 1994). However, a 6–8 week trial is often recommended to allow evaluation of the persistence of the therapeutic effects. With some compounds, such as clomipramine–a tricyclic antidepressant that has demonstrated efficacy in Obsessive Compulsive Disorder–patients have not shown improvement until the fourth to sixth week of treatment (Grof et al., 1993). It should be noted that in studies requiring titration to reach a maintenance dose, the titration period should not be counted as part of the four (or more) weeks of the trial.

Clinical trials of patients with acute schizophrenia will typically be short-term, placebo-controlled, inpatient studies lasting approximately 4–8 weeks. In recent years, however, there has been some discussion by the FDA's Psychopharmacologic Drugs Advisory Committee on decreasing the duration to two weeks, as differences between active treatments and placebo can generally be detected within this amount of time (Sramek et al., 1997). Longer exposures could then be evaluated using more stable patients for up to one year or more, randomly assigned to the study medication or a reference antipsychotic compound. Because of the known risks of relapse in unmedicated schizophrenic patients (Davis, 1985), such trials generally should not include a placebo arm.

Compounds for the treatment of Alzheimer's disease (AD) require much longer clinical trials, on the scale of months to years. The benefits of longer trials are readily apparent, as the magnitude of differences between placebo- and drug-treated patients often increases with the duration of the trial (Davis, 1996). A six-month trial is recommended to detect placebo-drug differences with symptomatic treatments such as acetylcholinesterase inhibitors. As many new compounds are designed to slow the progression of the disease, rather than just treat symptoms, trials of 1–2 years or more might be necessary to detect beneficial effects.

As most psychotropic drugs are used for prolonged periods of time, it has been suggested that data concerning maintenance effects are lacking in most clinical development programs. Klein (1991) has noted that some drugs that have gained approval have been reported to work for a short period of time before failing. Moreover, there is generally little information available concerning how long patients should be kept on the medication in order to minimize the risk of relapse. Thus, although trials evaluating the maintenance effects of investigational compounds require a duration of approximately 6–12 months, the information gained could be crucial to the optimal clinical use of the compound.

MUST EVERY TRIAL BE A PLACEBO-CONTROLLED, DOUBLE-BLIND, PARALLEL GROUP DESIGN?

Regulatory Guidelines

Specifically, the FDA guidelines on 'adequate and well-controlled' studies require that the design of a clinical trial permit a valid comparison of the investigational compound with a control, in order to provide a

BOX 4.1 FIVE TYPES OF CONTROLLED TRIALS

Placebo concurrent control. The test drug is compared with an inactive preparation designed to resemble the test drug as much as possible. A placebo-controlled study may include additional treatment groups, such as an active treatment control or a dose-comparison control, and usually includes a randomization and blinding of patients or investigators, or both.

Dose-comparison concurrent control. At least two doses of the drug are compared. A dose-comparison study may include additional treatment groups, such as placebo control or active control. Dose-comparison trials usually include randomization and blinding of patients or investigators, or both.

No treatment concurrent control. Where objective measurements of effectiveness are available and placebo effect is negligible, the test drug is compared with no treatment. No treatment concurrent control trials usually include randomization.

Active treatment concurrent control. The test drug is compared with a known effective therapy; for example, where the condition treated is such that administration of a placebo or no treatment would be contrary to the interest of the patient. An active treatment study may include additional treatment groups, however, such as placebo control or a dose-comparison control. Active treatment trials usually include randomization and blinding of patients or investigators, or both. If the intent of the trial is to show similarity of the test and control drugs, the report of the study should assess the ability of the study to have detected a difference between treatments. Similarity of the test drug and active control can mean either that both drugs were effective or that neither was effective. The analysis of the study should explain why the drugs should be considered effective in the study, for example, by reference to results in previous placebo-controlled studies of the active control drug.

Historical control: The results of treatment with the test drug are compared with experience historically derived from the adequately documented natural history of the disease or condition, or from the results of active treatment, in comparable patients or populations. Because historical control populations usually cannot be assessed with respect to pertinent variables as well as concurrent control populations, historical control designs are usually reserved for special circumstances. Examples include studies of diseases with high and predictable mortality (for example, certain malignancies) and studies in which the effect of the drug is self-evident (general anesthetics, drug metabolism).

21 Code of Federal Regulations, 314.126

quantitative assessment of the drug effect. These guidelines recognize five general types of controlled trials that are considered to be capable of satisfying the requirements of an adequate and well-controlled investigation in Phase II/III (Box 4.1). However, the appropriateness of each type of design is dependent upon the clinical condition under study.

For the purposes of gaining FDA approval, the use of a placebo concurrent control or an active treatment concurrent control is clearly necessary to provide compelling evidence of efficacy in CNS indications. However, the question of which of these two designs is most appropriate has both scientific and ethical implications.

The use of an active treatment control relies on the assumption that the outcome of a trial is the result of the pharmacological effects of the compounds administered, rather than outside influences. This assumption could be inaccurate, particularly in the case of CNS indications which can resolve spontaneously or fluctuate in intensity (Leber, 1991). For example, Leber (1991) documented the potential hazards of relying on active treatment controls in an analysis of six randomized controlled trials submitted in a new drug application (NDA) for a novel antidepressant. In each of these studies, patients were randomized to receive the investigational compound, doses of imipramine considered adequate to treat outpatients with depression, or placebo. A statistical comparison of patients treated with imipramine and the investigational compound strongly suggested that improvement was similar between the two groups, implying that the new drug was not only effective, but equipotent to imipramine. However, when the outcome of the patients receiving placebo was taken into consideration, only one of the six studies supported the antidepressant efficacy of the investigational compound. Without the placebo arm, these studies would have wrongfully assumed that the improvement of the two active treatment groups was due to the pharmacological effects of the compounds administered.

However, while placebo-controlled studies are more likely to control for outside influences, such as spontaneous change in disease course or biased observation, some researchers have questioned the ethical acceptability of administering placebo to patients where standard alternative therapies exist. This issue is particularly important in disorders such as schizophrenia and severe depression, where patients could be put at risk for psychosis or suicide when taken off of their regular medication. Thus, the risks associated with the administration of placebo must be weighed against the risk of conducting a study that is methodologically unsound. The ethical issues of placebo controls are discussed in more detail later in this chapter.

Although regulatory requirements do not specifically require all studies to be placebo-controlled, randomized, and double-blind, uncontrolled studies or partially controlled studies cannot be used as the sole basis for drug approval.   Instead, these studies are used as corroborative evidence supporting the efficacy of the investigational compound, or to provide additional information useful in the evaluation of an optimal dose regimen.   Here, a distinction must be drawn between studies that are intended to be used for the regulatory purposes of approval versus those that are intended to gain complementary medical or scientific knowledge.   Blinded, randomized, controlled studies are still considered to be the gold standard as the primary basis for determining whether there is 'substantial evidence' of efficacy.

Alternative Study Designs

The optimal design for a clinical trial is determined by the nature of the question under investigation. Thus, traditional, placebo-controlled, double-blind, parallel-group studies are not likely to be useful for all types of investigations, and the advent of new treatment strategies could prompt a need for innovative trial designs.   An example of this situation is the development of new drugs for the treatment of AD.

In drug development for the treatment of AD, the focus has recently shifted from the alleviation of symptoms to the slowing or prevention of the disease process. However, the evaluation of compounds designed to affect disease progression has implications for clinical trial design.   While traditional, placebo-controlled, double-blind, parallel group studies have been instrumental in evaluating the efficacy of investigational compounds against the symptoms of AD, the question of how to differentiate symptomatic benefit from a slowing of disease progression have not yet been answered.

Recently, Leber (1996) proposed two alternative study designs for clinical trials of AD compounds, intended to distinguish symptomatic from disease-altering effects. The first design is based on the concept of drug withdrawal. The premise for this approach is that a treatment affecting only the symptoms of the disease should produce its beneficial effects only during drug administration without persisting after the drug is withdrawn. In contrast, a drug that results in beneficial effects due to an alteration of the disease process itself should maintain these benefits even when the drug is withdrawn. While some deterioration is still expected after withdrawal of the drug, the relative benefits over patients receiving placebo should remain constant.

However, there are several methodological issues which must be resolved before such a trial can be undertaken. For example, how long should the patients be followed after withdrawal from the study drug? How can the problem of attrition be resolved? Additionally, there is the ethical issue of withdrawing patients from a treatment which could provide substantial beneficial effects. To address these factors, Leber (1996) proposed an alternative 'randomized start design' in which patients do not have to be withdrawn from the investigational treatment. This design consists of two distinct phases. In the first phase, patients are randomized to receive either active treatment or placebo, an identical design to the traditional, randomized, parallel-group, placebo-controlled study. At the end of the first phase, however, patients in the placebo group are switched to active treatment so that all patients are now receiving the same regimen. The two groups then continue to receive the investigational compound through the duration of the second phase of the study.

In order for this design to provide useful information, there must be a statistically significant difference between the two treatment groups at the end of the first phase of the study which demonstrates beneficial effects in patients receiving the active treatment. At this point, the improvement in the active treatment group could be attributed to either symptomatic or disease-altering effects. However, the relative improvement of patients initially randomized to receive placebo in the second phase of the study will be indicative of whether the active treatment group experienced symptomatic or disease-altering effects. If we assume that the benefits of the active drug were due to disease-altering processes, then the group randomized to placebo cannot be expected to make up for the structural losses they experienced while receiving placebo, even once they are administered the active drug. If the original placebo group improves in the second phase to the extent that they 'catch up' to the active treatment group, however, then one can assume that the improvements were due to an alleviation of symptoms.

Leber (1996) acknowledges some difficulties with the randomized start design, including the fact that a failure to find a difference at the end of the first phase will result in a failure of the study. There is also the likelihood that the results of the between-group comparison at the end of the first phase will not be known until after the second phase has begun. Additionally, this design does not address the potential outcome of untreated patients in the second phase of the study (to this end, Leber has suggested that a third, placebo-treated arm be included in the design).

However, the advantage of the randomized start design over the withdrawal design is clear, as no patients are required to be removed from an active treatment which they and their caregivers may believe is beneficial. This design is also much more capable of evaluating the disease-altering effects of new drugs than the traditional parallel-group design. Innovative ideas such as these will no doubt contribute to our understanding of the disease process and provide new options for clinical trial design in future studies.

Ethical Issues and Placebo Controls

A placebo has been defined as any therapy (or component of therapy) that is used for its nonspecific, psychological, or psychophysiological effects (Shapiro and Shapiro, 1984). Correspondingly, placebo effects are responses to a therapy that are unrelated to any known pharmacological action. An analysis of the literature reveals that placebo effects can be quite high in trials of psychotropic compounds. In moderate to severe depression, placebo response rates can range from 30–40%, increasing to over 50% for patients with less severe illness (Brown, 1988). Estimates of placebo effects in anxiety disorders vary widely, with a reported range of 18–67% in GAD (Loebel et al., 1986) and 22% in panic disorder (Black et al., 1993). Even in schizophrenia, where placebo response is generally considered to be low, a review of the literature on placebo-controlled studies in schizophrenia found that the percentage of placebo responders in short-term trials amounts to 0–40%, while the response rate is 40–60% with active treatment (Lewander, 1994). These numbers suggest that placebo effects are a potentially serious confound requiring internal control in efficacy studies.

There are two principal scientific incentives for using placebo controls. First, placebos can control for a multitude of nonspecific effects that could confound the evaluation of drug efficacy, including: the passage of time (particularly for disorders with a tendency to remit), increased attention and encouragement from clinical study staff, patient expectations and hope for improvement, and the psychosocial consequences of legitimization of the sick role (DeDeyn, 1995). Second, though equally important, is the ability of placebo controls to calibrate the skills of the clinical staff. The outcome and sensitivity of a study are highly reliant both upon the instruments that are used and the accuracy and reliability with which they are used (Addington et al., 1997).

However, it has been argued that the ethics of using placebos in psychotropic drug trials are questionable because patients are denied treatment with established compounds (Rothman and Michels, 1994). With the advent of increasingly effective standard treatments for many CNS disorders, the argument against placebo controls has become even more significant. However, evidence suggests that when used correctly, placebo controls are an ethical research tool. One important point is that in some indications with very high placebo response rates (such as depression or anxiety), the administration of a placebo is not equivalent to 'no treatment.' Indeed, the difference in improvement rates between drug-treated and placebo-treated patients is probably not large enough to render placebo control unethical for many patients with these indications (Sramek and Cutler, 1995; DeDeyn, 1995). The situation is more complicated for indications such as schizophrenia, where there is a risk of psychotic relapse. Thus, in trials of antipsychotics, it is imperative that patients are carefully monitored throughout the study, as well as an adequate follow-up period. Appropriate escape medication should also be provided, along with predetermined exit criteria designed to protect the welfare of the patients.

In trials of compounds for AD, there is a strong argument for the ethical use of placebo controls, as there is no true standard therapy at this time. Even tacrine, which has demonstrated efficacy in the treatment of this disease, was only shown to be clinically effective in 23% of patients with dementia of the Alzheimer's type (Knapp et al., 1994). Additionally, tacrine and many other cholinesterase inhibitors are not devoid of side effects, most notably the elevation of liver enzymes (Knapp et al., 1994). Finally, placebo administration does not appear to present an unacceptable risk to patients suffering from this slowly progressing neurodegenerative disorder (DeDeyn, 1995).

Arguments regarding the ethical acceptability of placebo controls are often the result of the apparently irreconcilable conflict between individuals who want immediate effective treatment, and a collective set of individuals (society), which wants to develop better treatments through scientific progress. If we were to adhere to the individual viewpoint, we would still be satisfied with the use of reserpine for schizophrenia, strophanthus for heart failure, or malariotherapy for syphilis, as these treatments were considered to be effective in our modern age of medicine (Goodman et al., 1985; Stolley, 1992). In fact, our latest treatments for these illnesses are still suboptimal. If we take the societal viewpoint, we can understand the rationale of pursuing new treatments even where effective ones exist. Nonetheless, the balance between the two viewpoints is a difficult one. In a free society, responsible and informed individuals formulate decisions on the behalf of others, not just striking a balance by compromising both positions, but by insuring that the benefits outweigh the risks.

Furthermore, there is the ethical obligation of the researcher to conduct scientifically sound studies. As investigators, we should be committed to preventing ineffective drugs from entering the marketplace. These ideas are echoed by the World Health Organization in its strong case for placebo-controlled trials:

> It is generally accepted that a drug evaluation can be considered ethical only if it is likely to provide information useful to patients... Thus, as commonly applied, only placebo-controlled evaluations have uniformly provided meaningful findings... Such considerations may support the use of placebo-controlled designs even in situations where efficacious treatments are available, for example in acutely ill psychotic patients...Thus, overall, the placebo alone or preferably in combination with a standard treatment control, is usually an essential instrument in the drug evaluation process. (11, p 28–9)

The earlier example by Leber (1991) demonstrates the potential for misleading results when a placebo control is not employed. As DeDeyn (1995) has stated, 'A methodologically bad trial is always unethical.'

Of course, the reverse of this statement is not true; that is, not every methodologically sound trial is ethical. There are clearly several issues which must be addressed when a placebo is used in a clinical trial, in order to ensure that patients are not put in a position of unacceptable risk. Improper dose selection can also result in all patients receiving essentially placebo, or the other extreme, doses that are too toxic. Thus, safety and tolerance studies conducted in the patient population prior to dose selection for efficacy studies ('bridging studies') can help to ensure that accurate doses are included. Patient selection for placebo-controlled trials should address the potential adverse effects of placebo on a case-by-case basis, and exclude all individuals thought to be at risk for violence or suicide; this is especially important in trials of antipsychotics and antidepressants. Additionally, patients must be informed, prior to the study, that they could receive placebo and not an active drug. Patients should also be monitored closely, and discontinued from the study if they experience an exacerbation of symptoms. If appropriate measures are taken, high scientific standards can be achieved without compromising the welfare of the patients.

SINGLE-SITE VERSUS MULTICENTER STUDIES

A common problem in conducting large, pivotal studies in a drug development program is recruiting adequate numbers of qualified patients. For this reason, most large, Phase III studies have employed a multicenter design, in which patients are enrolled at several distinct sites. This design allows investigators to take advantage of a much larger patient pool, and to carry out large-scale studies in a shorter period of time. Unfortunately, our experience with multicenter studies suggests that approximately one third of the sites provide efficient enrollment, one third lag behind, and one third fail to enroll adequate numbers of patients. Discrepancies in patient enrollment between sites has unfavorable consequences not only for timely study completion, but also for the statistical power to detect efficacy.

Perhaps even more serious is the variability that a multicenter study can introduce into the data. For example, the patient pool may be quite heterogeneous across various sites. This issue is of particular concern in cross-national studies, where ethnic and cultural differences add another dimension to the patient population. Additionally, the use of distinct investigational sites raises the possibility of differences in diagnostic standards, despite the use of standardized rating instruments. Although protocols generally specify standard rating scales, the potential for reduced inter-rater reliability becomes a concern as the number of raters and sites increases. Thus, the clean data obtained from a few of the sites could be obscured by the lackluster performance at the majority of sites.

The potential dangers of conducting a multicenter study are illustrated by a placebo-controlled trial of ipsapirone and lorazepam, in which the results from our single site (n = 90) are contrasted with the entire six-site study (n = 317). In our single-site study (Cutler et al., 1993a), we reported a mean reduction on the Hamilton Rating Scale for Anxiety (HAM-A) of 12.9 points for patients receiving ipsapirone, 11.0 points for patients receiving lorazepam, and 5.4 points for patients receiving placebo after completion of the acute treatment period. In the multicenter study (Cutler et al., 1993b), the mean reduction in HAM-A scores was 12.7 points for patients receiving ipsapirone, 11.7 points for patients receiving lorazepam, and 9.3 points for patients receiving placebo. While improvement on the HAM-A was similar for drug-treated patients in both studies, the placebo response in the multicenter study was nearly four points greater than the single-site study. The placebo response for the multicenter study is so high that when the results of our site are removed from the analysis, the difference between active drug and placebo fails to achieve statistical significance. Upon closer inspection, we noted that at one site, the three treatment groups demonstrated similar improvement (a reduction of approximately 15 points on the HAM-A) and that two other sites reported a greater improvement with placebo than with either ipsapirone or lorazepam. Thus, at half of the sites in the multicenter study, placebo was found to be equally effective or more effective than two established anxiolytic compounds. Placebo response rates of this magnitude have the potential to significantly delay drug development by rendering data that is inaccurate and unusable.

In a trial involving a smaller number of sites, the potential for more consistent rater training is increased. Thus, standard deviations in efficacy and safety ratings would be smaller than those found across several distinct sites. Furthermore, sponsoring pharmaceutical companies could complete study monitoring in a more convenient and timely manner in a study with fewer sites. Previous studies have shown that planning and coordinating multicenter studies while keeping quality control at a high level across multiple sites is a difficult prospect (Pocock, 1985). Due to the additional travel and start-up costs, multicenter trials also tend to cost more. Thus, conducting a trial with one or two experienced, capable sites could save both time and money.

REFERENCES

Addington D, Williams R, Lapierre Y, el-Guebaly N. Placebos in clinical trials of psychotropic medication. *Can J Psychiatry* 1997; **42**(3): 6.

Black DW, Wesner R, Bowers W, Gabel J. A comparison of fluvoxamine, cognitive therapy and placebo in the treatment of panic disorder. *Arch Gen Psychiatry* 1993; **50**(1): 44–50.

Brown WA. Predictors of placebo response in depression. *Psychopharmacol Bull* 1988; **24**: 14–17.

Cutler NR, Sramek JJ, Keppel-Hesselink JM, et al. A double-blind, placebo-controlled study comparing the efficacy and safety of ipsapirone versus lorazepam in patients with generalized anxiety disorder: a prospective multicenter trial. *J Clin Psychopharmacol* 1993a; **13**: 429–437.

Cutler NR, Sramek JJ, Kurtz NM. Anxiolytic Compounds: Perspectives in Drug Development. Chichester, England: John Wiley & Sons, 1994.

Cutler NR, Sramek JJ, Wardle TS et al. The safety and efficacy of ipsapirone versus lorazepam in outpatients with generalized anxiety disorder (GAD): single site findings from a multicenter trial. *Psychopharmacol Bull* 1993b; **29**: 303–308.

Davis JM. Maintenance therapy and the natural course of schizophrenia. *J Clin Psychiatry* 1985; **46**: 18–21.

Davis KL. Issues in accelerating the pace of development for neuroprotective agents. *Alzheimer Dis Assoc Disord* 1996; **10**(1): 36–37.

DeDeyn PP. On the ethical acceptability of placebo application in neuropsychiatric research. *Acta Neurol Belg* 1995; **95**(1): 8–17.

Goodman AG, Gilman LS, Rall TW, Muraf F, eds. *Goodman and Gilman's The Pharmacological Basis of Therapeutics*, 7th ed. New York: MacMillan Pubs., 1985.

Grof P, Akhter MI, Campbell M, et al. *Clinical Evaluation of Psychotropic Drugs and Psychiatric Disorders.* Seattle: Hogrefe & Huber, 1993.

Klein DF. Improvement of phase III psychotropic drug trials by intensive phase II work. *Neuropsychopharmacology* 1991; **4**(4): 251–258.

Knapp MJ, Knopman D, Solomon PR, Pendlebury WW, Davis CS, Gracon SI. A 30-week randomized controlled trial of high-dose tacrine in patients with Alzheimer's disease. *JAMA* 1994; **271**: 985–991.

Leber P. Is there an alternative to the randomized controlled trial? *Psychopharmacol Bull* 1991; **27**(1): 3–8.

Leber P. Observations and suggestions on antidementia drug development. *Alzheimer Dis Assoc Disord* 1996; **10**(Suppl 1): 31–35.

Lewander T. Placebo response in schizophrenia. *Eur Psychiatry* 1994; **9**: 119–120.

Loebel A, Hyde TS, Dunner DL. Early placebo response in anxious and depressed patients. *J Clin Psychiatry* 1986; **47**: 230–232.

Pocock SJ. Current issues in the design and interpretation of clinical trials. *Br Med J* 1985; **290**: 39–42.

Quitkin FM, Rabkin JG, Ross D, McGrath PJ. Duration of antidepressant drug treatment. *Arch Gen Psychiatry* 1984; **41**: 238–245.

Rothman KJ, Michels KB. The unethical use of placebo controls. *N Eng J Med* 1994; **331**: 394–397.

Shapiro AK, Shapiro E. Patient-provider relationships and the placebo effect. In: Metarazzo JD, Weiss SM, Herd JA, Miller NE (eds) *Behavioral Health: A Handbook of Health Enhancement and Disease Prevention.* New York: Wiley-Interscience, 1984.

Sramek JJ, Cutler NR. The use of placebo controls [letter, comment]. *N Engl J Med* 1995; **332**(1): 62.

Sramek JJ, Cutler NR, Kurtz NM, Murphy MF, Carta A. Optimizing the Development of Antipsychotic Drugs. Chichester, England: John Wiley & Sons, 1997.

Sramek JJ, Jasinsky O, Chang S, Shu V, Kashkin K, Kennedy S, Sadd C, Cutler NR. Pilot efficacy trial of ABT-200 in patients with major depressive disorder. *Depression* 1994/1995; **2**: 315–318.

Stolley P. Shortcuts in drug evaluation. *Clin Pharm Ther* 1992; **32**:1–3.

5   The bridging study: Optimizing the dose for Phase II/III

REVIEW OF CLINICAL TRIAL DESIGN

Traditional drug development consists of four phases of clinical testing in humans. The primary goal of *Phase I* studies is to evaluate the safety and tolerability of the investigational drug in a small number of healthy volunteers, and to determine the optimal dose range for later studies. This phase also includes studies of pharmacokinetic measures in order to determine drug metabolism and bioavailability.

Phase II studies estimate the preliminary efficacy of the drug in a relatively small number of patients in order to determine if large-scale comparative trials are warranted. Phase II studies are often dose-finding studies which attempt to identify the dose range at which beneficial effects are most likely to occur without prohibitive side effects.

If a compound demonstrates efficacy in Phase II, *Phase III* studies will test the drug in larger groups of patients in order to verify efficacy and determine whether any side effects are associated with long-term use. In Phase III, the strict inclusion/exclusion criteria employed in Phase II are often relaxed to include a wider range of patient characteristics than previously allowed, as more information about the safety profile of the compound becomes available. On occasion, however, the criteria may be stricter if specific adverse events are identified. Phase III studies will also generally employ a placebo or active control group.

Phase IV studies are designed to evaluate factors not fully explored in previous phases. These factors can include the effects of a compound in special patient populations or its potential use in other indications. For example, the New Drug Application for the antipsychotic risperidone did not have adequate information on drug effects in elderly patients, thus requiring further study of this population. In addition to these studies, post-marketing surveillance is often performed in order to compile additional adverse event data from physicians who have prescribed the drug to their patients. A variety of dosing regimens and durations may also be compared for safety and efficacy.

Although the clinical evaluation process has remained largely unchanged over the past few decades, a desire to bring novel compounds to the marketplace faster and more economically has inspired some suggestions for accelerating early drug development. One solution is the 'bridging study,' in which a late Phase I (Ib) or early Phase II (IIa) safety/tolerance study is conducted directly in the patient population (Cutler et al., 1996; Cutler and Sramek, 1995a; Cutler and Sramek, 1995b). Traditionally, Phase I safety/tolerance studies have been conducted in healthy volunteers for several reasons, including medical-legal complications associated with patients, concerns for their safety, and issues of convenience (Weissman, 1981). However, there is evidence that patients tolerate certain CNS compounds differently than healthy subjects, and that Phase I studies in normals can be poorly predictive of the optimal dose range for Phase II studies in the target population.

PATIENTS VS. HEALTHY SUBJECTS

Differences in drug response between patients and healthy subjects are not surprising, as most CNS compounds affect neurotransmitter or receptor systems that are altered in the target population. For example, several studies have reported that schizophrenic patients tolerate higher doses of antipsychotic compounds than healthy controls (Figure 5.1). Okuma (1981) found that schizophrenic patients demonstrated a quantitatively lower sensitivity to the sedative effects of chlorpromazine than healthy volunteers, as demonstrated by a higher percent time of waking EEG following dose administration. Miller et al. (1993) reported that a significantly higher percentage of normal subjects experienced dystonia/tremor, restlessness, sedation, and anticholinergic side effects following the acute administration of haloperidol. The difference in sensitivity was attributed to higher dopamine receptor levels in schizophrenic patients, resulting in less complete dopaminergic blockade following the neuroleptic challenge. Another potential mechanism for the difference in tolerability is an increased post-synaptic dopamine receptor sensitivity in schizophrenic patients (Owen et al., 1978). In one early haloperidol study in which normal male volunteers were given up to 5 mg as a single dose, most of the volunteers needed to be rushed to an emergency room for treatment of

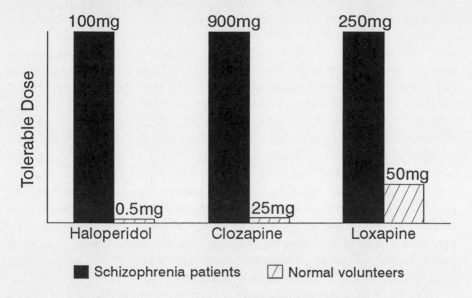

Figure 5.1 Differences in antipsychotic drug tolerance between schizophrenic patients and normal volunteers. Reproduced by permission from Sramek et al., 1997.

severe and serious reactions, including laryngeal dystonia (G.M. Simpson, personal communication).

Differences in antipsychotic tolerance between patients and healthy subjects are not limited to dopamine D_2 receptor antagonists. In a recent study in which 17 healthy male subjects were administered single 25 mg doses of clozapine (Clozaril®), eight of the subjects experienced severe bradycardia (< 40 bpm), and two of these subjects had cardiac arrest lasting 10 and 60 seconds, respectively (Pokorny et al., 1994). Although all subjects recovered, a recommendation was made by the FDA that future bioequivalence studies of clozapine be conducted only in schizophrenic patients.

Patients have also demonstrated a higher tolerance than healthy subjects for benzodiazepines and tricyclic antidepressants (Grof et al., 1993). Many patients with GAD can tolerate up to 30 mg of diazepam per day, while healthy subjects would be likely to experience extreme sedation at this dose. Additionally, in a recent study of the novel anxiolytic, lesopitron, we found that patients with GAD were able to tolerate considerably higher doses than healthy subjects (Sramek et al., 1996a). This study will be discussed in more detail later in the chapter.

In our experience with clinical trials of compounds for the treatment of Alzheimer's disease (AD), we have found that patients often tolerate higher doses than healthy elderly subjects, but can sometimes tolerate only lower doses (Cutler et al., 1994; Cutler et al., 1995). Additionally, in a recent study, Medina et al. (1997) reported that AD patients demonstrated a reduced risk of tilt-induced syncope following the oral administration of xanomeline in comparison to healthy, age-matched controls. This result suggests that patients may have a lower susceptibility to the cardiovascular effects of M_1-receptor stimulation, presumably due to the lower muscarinic receptor activity associated with AD.

The importance of determining differences in tolerance between healthy subjects and the target patient population is illustrated by the potential dose-response relationships of an investigational compound (Figure 5.2). For the majority of CNS-active compounds, both treatment response and toxicity tend to increase linearly with dose. Although compounds with more complex receptor pharmacology can sometimes demonstrate more complicated dose-response relationships, this general trend suggests that the potential to detect efficacy is enhanced at the highest

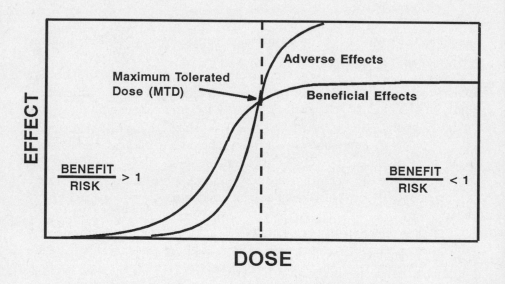

Figure 5.2 Example of a dose-response relationship

tolerable doses of a compound. If patients are able to tolerate higher doses of a compound than healthy subjects, conducting a bridging study prior to Phase II could help researchers to avoid selecting a dose range that is too low, thus optimizing the chances of detecting efficacy. Conversely, if patients can tolerate only lower doses of a compound, a bridging study could enhance the safety of Phase II by avoiding selection of a dose range that is too high.

METHODOLOGY OF THE BRIDGING STUDY

In a bridging study, consecutive panels of patients each receive higher doses of study drug until a minimum intolerated dose (MID) is reached. The MID can be defined as the dose at which 50% of patients experience severe or multiple moderate adverse events probably related to the study drug, or one patient experiences a serious adverse event (defined as medically unacceptable) believed to be related to the study drug. The dose immediately below this one is the maximum tolerated dose (MTD). One important point, however, is that the definition of what is medically unacceptable might differ depending on the population under study. For example, what is considered unacceptable for a healthy subject might not be so for a patient with a chronic illness. Thus, indication-specific prospective criteria should be identified prior to initiation of a trial, in order to determine an accurate MTD.

The design of a bridging study is somewhat dependent upon the particular compound under investigation. Generally, bridging studies for AD compounds employ a fixed-dose panel design, in which consecutive panels of 6–8 patients each receive doses that range from 50% below to 50% or more above the MTD in healthy subjects for (see Table 5.1). Each of the consecutive panels is dependent on the tolerability of the previous dose level. The dose level is increased until the MID is reached; the dose immediately preceding the MID is designated the MTD.

In some cases, it is beneficial to conclude the study with titration of a final panel in order to determine any differences in tolerability between fixed and titrated doses, as titration may re-define the MTD. An example of a titration panel design is shown in Table 5.2.

In order to maximize the safety of the bridging study, we recommend exploring the animal toxicology of the study compound at dosages beyond anticipated human dosages to provide the best possible understanding of potential adverse events, and taking care with subject selection (Cutler et

Table 5.1 Bridging study: a recommended fixed-dose design

Fixed-dose panel design: inpatient assessment

Panel 1: 50% less than MTD

Panel 2: 25% less than MTD

Panel 3: MTD based on healthy normals

Panel 4: 25% greater than MTD

Panel 5: 50% greater than MTD[a]

[a] Study may require panels with higher doses to define the MTD

al., 1994 and 1996; Cutler and Sramek, 1995a and 1995b). Patients should be in good physical health, with no significant concurrent medical disease. Additionally, phenotyping for drug metabolizing enzymes could be beneficial for understanding and correlating responses of poor and extensive metabolizers to the investigational compound.

As bridging studies examine doses at the high end of the tolerability spectrum, they should be conducted only in facilities with hospital-quality intensive care equipment and qualified critical care nurses and physicians. In order to minimize patient discomfort or risk, rigorous and careful supervision is required. Patients should be monitored closely and questioned frequently in order to avoid the possibility that negative experiences will go unreported. In previous bridging studies we have

Table 5.2 Bridging study: a recommended titration design

Titration panel doses: inpatient assessment	Duration
50% less than MTD	x 4 days
25% less than MTD	x 4 days
Fixed-dose MTD in patients	x 4 days
25% greater than MTD	x 4 days
50% greater than MTD	x 4 days

conducted, a panel of six patients is attended by no fewer than two critical care nurses in addition to ancillary nursing staff (as necessary) on a 24-hour basis (Cutler and Sramek, 1995a).

EXAMPLES OF BRIDGING STUDIES IN ALZHEIMER'S DISEASE

Our first experiences with bridging involved the evaluation of compounds for the treatment of AD, including several acetylcholinesterase inhibitors and muscarinic agonists. Through these studies, bridging methodology evolved into the designs that are outlined in the previous section. In addition, the results of these studies emphasized the value of determining the MTD in the target patient population prior to the selection of a dose range for Phase II/III efficacy studies.

Velnacrine

Velnacrine (HP 029) is a centrally acting acetylcholinesterase inhibitor that has demonstrated efficacy in animal models of memory loss (Jackson et al., 1995). In a previous, single-dose study in healthy young male volunteers (n = 70), doses up to 200 mg were generally well tolerated. One subject experienced dizziness, loose stools, vomiting, and moderate headache at 75 mg, and another subject reported moderate headache at 200 mg (Puri et al., 1989). A single-dose, double-blind, placebo-controlled, inpatient study of 50–300 mg velnacrine was also conducted in healthy elderly subjects (n = 45). Lower doses (50 and 100 mg) were well tolerated; however, minor gastrointestinal adverse events were observed at doses of 150 and 200 mg. All subjects in the 300 mg dose group experienced adverse events such as gastrointestinal cramps, nausea, vomiting, and diarrhea. Thus, 100 mg was designated the highest well-tolerated dose (Puri et al., 1988).

An ascending, multiple-dose, double-blind, placebo-controlled study of velnacrine was then conducted in 56 healthy, elderly male subjects. Doses of 25, 50, and 100 mg administered twice daily (BID) or 100 mg administered three times daily (TID) were evaluated for 28 days. Gastrointestinal adverse events were observed at doses of 100 mg BID and TID; however, the majority of these events were reported during the initial nine days of dosing and did not recur. Although no higher doses were evaluated, 100 mg TID was designated the MTD (Puri et al., 1990).

Our bridging study was designed to evaluate the safety and tolerability of velnacrine at doses up to 450 mg in patients with AD (Cutler et al., 1990). A total of 24 patients (12 males, 12 females, mean age 73 years) participated in this double-blind, placebo-controlled, dose-escalation study in three groups of eight patients each. In each group, 6 patients were randomized to receive velnacrine and 2 patients were randomized to receive placebo for 10 days. Patients were required to meet NINCDS-ADRDA criteria for AD, and to have a Mini-Mental State Examination (MMSE) score between 10 and 26. Patients were to be free of medical, neurological, or psychiatric disease, or any other conditions which could interfere with the absorption, distribution, or excretion of the study drug.

Patients in Group 1 were to receive placebo or velnacrine, titrated to doses of 450 mg (administered TID). However, velnacrine was poorly tolerated, with patients experiencing nausea, vomiting, abdominal pain, dizziness, and syncope. One patient had a clonic/tonic seizure approximately 6 h after the second 150 mg dose, following protracted nausea, vomiting, and hyperventilation, and was discontinued from the study. Thus, Group 1 was discontinued on Day 5, and the maximum doses for Groups 2 and 3 were reduced.

In Group 2, velnacrine-treated patients received titrated doses up to 300 mg. At 300 mg, four of the six patients receiving velnacrine were discontinued from the study due to severe adverse events including headache, dizziness, and fainting. Nausea and vomiting were also reported in these patients. The maximum dose for Group 3 was thus set at 225 mg.

In Group 3, velnacrine was well tolerated at doses up to 225 mg. Mild adverse events, including nausea, vomiting, lacrimation, and rhinorrhea, occurred in only two patients receiving active drug. No patients in any group demonstrated clinically significant changes in vital signs, clinical lab values, or ECG measures during the study. Thus, 225 mg was considered the MTD in AD patients.

This study highlights the importance of patient selection in the bridging study, as the response of a single patient could determine the decision for further dose escalation. Additionally, the rate of titration should also be considered, as a slower titration might have increased MTD of velnacrine through the development of tolerance.

In conclusion, our bridging study found that AD patients tolerated lower doses of velnacrine than both healthy young and elderly subjects. The MTD in patients was 25% lower than the highest well-tolerated dose (300 mg) in healthy elderly subjects.

Eptastigmine

An earlier study of eptastigmine evaluated the safety and tolerability of single doses of 4, 8, 20, and 40 mg in healthy young subjects (n = 19). Lower doses of 4–20 mg were well tolerated, with subjects reporting mild adverse events such as headache and fatigue. Severe, dose-limiting adverse events including nausea, blurred vision, dizziness, headache, symptomatic orthostatic hypotension, and palpitations associated with sinus tachycardia were observed at 40 mg (Goldberg et al., 1991). In another study, eight healthy elderly subjects received eptastigmine at doses of 8, 20, 32, and 40 mg. Again, dose-limiting adverse events such as nausea, vomiting, and headache were observed at 40 mg. In this study, 32 mg was designated the MTD.

We conducted a multiple-dose, two-phase, double-blind, placebo-controlled bridging study (Sramek et al., 1995a) in 20 patients with AD (12 males, eight females, mean age 74 years). Patients were diagnosed with probable AD according to NINCDS-ADRDA and DSM-III-R criteria, and were required to be free of any medical, neurological, or psychiatric disorders, or any abnormalities which could interfere with study assessments.

In the first phase of the study, three cohorts of patients received placebo or eptastigmine at ascending fixed doses of 12 mg TID (n = 4), 20 mg TID (n = 8), or 28 mg TID (n = 8) for 14 days. In each cohort, 25% of the patients received placebo. Progression to the next dose level was contingent upon the tolerability of the previous dose. All patients completed the study period without experiencing intolerable or severe adverse events.

Because no MTD was determined, an escalating dose phase was conducted in five patients who had received placebo in the fixed-dose phase. Patients were titrated from 28 mg TID to 48 mg TID, with dose increases of 4 mg TID every three days. Doses were then increased again by 4 mg TID every four days to a potential maximum dose of 56 mg TID. One patient in this phase received placebo.

In the titration phase, doses less than 48 mg TID were generally well tolerated. The most common adverse events in patients receiving eptastigmine were fatigue, agitation, nausea, and loose stools. After three days at 48 mg, one patient experienced severe dizziness, ataxia, and muscle cramps and was discontinued from the study. The study was terminated at 52 mg, when one patient experienced severe increased urinary frequency, a severe fall, and moderate bradykinesia, and another reported moderate somnolence. All adverse events were transient, and no clinically significant abnormalities were observed on ECG or laboratory tests at the end of the study.

Due to the severe adverse events observed in two patients at 52 mg TID, 48 mg TID was designated the MTD in this study. Thus, the MTD in AD patients was 50% higher than the highest tolerated dose in healthy elderly subjects.

SDZ ENA 713

SDZ ENA 713 is a centrally active acetylcholinesterase inhibitor of the carbamate type. SDZ ENA 713 has demonstrated more potent AChE inhibition in cortex and hippocampus (both targets for symptomatic treatment of AD) than in other brain areas, and has shown a longer duration of cholinesterase blockade than tacrine (Enz et al., 1993). Early safety/tolerability studies of SDZ ENA 713 in healthy volunteers reported that multiple doses up to 3 mg/day were well tolerated. Doses of up to 3 mg BID were well tolerated in studies conducted in healthy elderly volunteers. Adverse events, including headache, dizziness, nausea, and diarrhea, were generally mild in intensity and were not dose-limiting. In an initial, placebo-controlled efficacy trial of SDZ ENA 713 in 402 AD patients, doses of 2 and 3 mg BID did not result in significant treatment effects after 13 weeks.

Our double-blind, placebo-controlled, parallel-group bridging study was designed to determine the MTD of SDZ ENA 713 in AD patients in order to maximize the potential for detecting efficacy in subsequent efficacy trials (Sramek et al., 1996b). Patients were required to meet NINCDS-ADRDA criteria for probable AD and to have an MMSE score between 10 and 26. Patients were excluded if they had any medical, neurological, or psychiatric disorders which could confound safety evaluations.

A total of 50 patients (22 males, 28 females, mean age 68 years) were randomized to receive SDZ ENA 713 BID (n = 20), SDZ ENA 713 TID (n = 20), or placebo (n = 10). Escalating doses for both SDZ ENA 713 treatment groups are shown in Table 5.3. If a dose was poorly tolerated, patients were allowed to skip up to six doses at each dose level, but no more than three in sequence. Three patients receiving SDZ ENA 713 discontinued from the study due to adverse events. One of these patients experienced a mild atrial fibrillation after receiving SDZ ENA 713 4 mg/day (TID regimen) and withdrew from the study; this event was later judged to be unrelated to study medication. The second patient began

Table 5.3 Bridging study of SDZ ENA 713: Dose-escalation schedule

Study Days/Week (s)	Dose
Days 1–3	2 mg/day
Days 4–7	3 mg/day
Week 2	4 mg/day
Week 3	5 mg/day
Week 4	6 mg/day
Week 5	7.25 mg/day
Week 6	8.5 mg/day
Week 7	10 mg/day
Weeks 8–9	12 mg/day

experiencing intermittent mild to moderate nausea and vomiting at 5 mg/day from the study after experiencing nausea and severe vomiting at 12 mg/day (TID regimen).

The most common adverse events reported for patients receiving SDZ ENA 713 were headache, nausea, dizziness, diarrhea, vomiting, and fatigue. Except for the patients who prematurely discontinued, adverse events associated with SDZ ENA 713 were generally transient and did not recur at higher doses. Thus, all doses were considered to be well tolerated, and no MTD was determined. Further doses were not explored, as 12 mg/day was the highest dose felt to be safe based on the preclinical No Observed Adverse Effect Level (NOAEL). Although this study did not reach an MTD, it extended the functional dose range well beyond the highest tolerated single dose in healthy subjects (3 mg/day). The evaluation of higher doses appears to have been advantageous in the development of SDZ ENA 713, as preliminary evidence from ongoing studies indicates that beneficial effects in patients with AD have been observed at doses of 3–12 mg/day (Anand and Hartman, 1996).

Metrifonate

Metrifonate is an organophosphorus compound which has previously been used in the treatment of schistosomiasis. Oral administration of metrifonate results in sustained acetylcholinesterase inhibition in both humans and animals (Hinz et al., 1996; Unni et al., 1994), and is associated with improved cognitive performance in animal models of memory loss (Itoh et al., 1997a, b; Riekkinen et al., 1997). In two previous studies, maintenance doses up to 0.65 mg/kg were generally well tolerated in healthy elderly volunteers, and maintenance doses of up to 1 mg/kg were well tolerated in AD patients (data on file, Bayer Corporation).

Our open-label bridging study was designed to evaluate the safety and tolerability of higher doses of metrifonate in two panels of patients (n = 8 per panel) with probable AD. In the first panel, patients received daily loading doses of 2.5 mg/kg for 14 days followed by 4 mg/kg for three days, with a subsequent daily maintenance dose of 2 mg/kg for 14 days. Patients were hospitalized during Study Days 15–24.

The initial loading dose phase was well tolerated, with the majority of adverse events reported as mild and transient. The most common adverse events were muscle cramps and abdominal discomfort. Although the incidence of gastrointestinal adverse events increased during the second loading dose phase, the tolerability profile of metrifonate initially improved with maintenance dosing. However, after four days at the maintenance dose, six of eight patients complained of generalized, moderate to severe weakness, the inability to resume daily activities, and difficulties with coordination. One patient with severe muscle weakness was hospitalized for observation and discontinued from the study. This incident was considered a serious adverse event, and the panel was terminated. All adverse events resolved after the discontinuation of metrifonate.

Due to the poor tolerability of the first panel, the original doses for the second panel were reduced. Patients in the second panel received a loading dose of 2.5 mg/kg for 14 days, followed by a maintenance dose of 1.5 mg/kg for 14 days. Patients were hospitalized during Study Days 21–23 and 47–49. Metrifonate was well tolerated during the loading dose phase, with patients reporting mild to moderate muscle cramps and gastrointestinal symptoms such as nausea, flatulence, and diarrhea. In the maintenance dose phase, one patient reported moderate diaphoresis, dizziness, and palpitations followed by severe intermittent abdominal cramps and tenderness. Due to these adverse events, this patient was hospitalized and prematurely discontinued from the study. Overall, the most common adverse events during the maintenance phase were gastrointestinal symptoms, muscle cramps, lightheadedness, and orthostatic hypotension. Most adverse events were reported to be transient and mild in intensity.

Thus, this bridging study defined 1.5 mg/kg as the MTD of metrifonate in AD patients. This maintenance dose substantially greater than the highest doses previously evaluated in healthy elderly subjects or in AD patients.

CI-979

CI-979 is a muscarinic agonist designed to provide cholinomimetic activity without excessive peripheral cholinergic effects. CI-979 has demonstrated central activity in preclinical studies of cognitive dysfunction, including reduction of spatial memory deficits induced by cortical lesions (Davis et al., 1993). In a previous study of CI-979 in 18 healthy young subjects, groups of six subjects each (four active drug; 2 placebo) were assigned to receive doses of 0.5, 1, or 2 mg q.6h for 14 days. Doses of 1 mg q.6h were considered well tolerated, with patients experiencing mild to moderate adverse events such as hypersalivation, chills, abdominal pain, increased perspiration, blurred vision, and increased urinary frequency. However, at the highest dose (2 mg q.6h) patients experienced severe, dose-limiting gastrointestinal adverse events, including abdominal cramps, vomiting, diarrhea, and nausea. Thus, 1 mg q.6h was designated the MTD for healthy young subjects in this study (Reece et al., 1992).

We conducted a rising, multiple-dose, double-blind, placebo-controlled, inpatient bridging study (Sramek et al., 1995b) in a single panel of 10 male AD patients (mean age 65 years). Patients met NINCDS-ADRDS and DSM-III-R criteria for AD, and had MMSE scores between 10 and 26. They had no clinically significant medical, neurological, or psychiatric disorders, or any conditions which could interfere with study evaluations.

Patients were randomized to receive placebo (n = 2) or rising doses of CI-979 (n = 8) for a period of 15 days. Doses were to be 0.5 mg q.6h, 1 mg q.12h, 1 mg q.6h, 2 mg q.12h, and 2 mg q.6h, administered sequentially for three days each. Dose escalation was contingent upon the absence of significant adverse events at lower doses. Five patients receiving CI-979 were prematurely discontinued from the study due to adverse events. Two patients discontinued after receiving 2 mg q.6h; one patient experienced mild postural hypotension, dizziness, hypersalivation, chills, nausea, and moderate diaphoresis, and another patient reported moderate Parkinsonian symptoms (bradykinesia, cogwheeling, gait, and tremor) as well as nausea, sweating, chills, hypersalivation, and dysuria. However, CI-979 was generally well tolerated by the remaining six patients, and the protocol was amended to include two additional doses of 2.5 mg q.6h for 1.5 days, and 3.0 mg q.6h for three days.

Two additional patients were withdrawn from the study after receiving CI-979 2.5 mg q.6h. One of these patients demonstrated severe Parkinsonian symptoms (cogwheeling, intention tremor, and pillrolling), was disoriented, and had hypersalivation, sweating, diarrhea, chills, rectal pain, and belching. The second patient complained of severe sweating, chills, coolness of the skin, moderate hypersalivation, and showed mild signs of parkinsonism (cogwheeling).

The frequency of adverse events increased with increasing dose. One further patient was discontinued after receiving 3 mg q.6h due to multiple episodes of moderate diarrhea, hypersalivation, sweating, and flatulence. The study was terminated at 3 mg q.6h due to multiple moderate cholinergic and gastrointestinal adverse events in three patients. Due to the severity of adverse events observed at 2.5 mg q.6h and 3 mg q.6h, 2 mg q.6h was designated the MTD in AD patients, a dose twice as high as the MTD found in healthy young subjects.

Xanomeline

Xanomeline tartrate is a potent and selective muscarinic agonist that has demonstrated high activity at cloned M_1 receptors (Shannon et al., 1994), and has been shown to cross the blood-brain barrier in man (Farde et al., 1993). In an escalating, single-dose study of xanomeline, the safety and tolerability of 1, 5, 10, 25, 50, 75, 100, and 150 mg were investigated in 36 young healthy subjects. Adverse events including diarrhea, diaphoresis, disorientation, increased diastolic blood pressure, nausea, and postural hypotension were observed at the 100 and 150 mg doses. A multiple-dose study of xanomeline reported that doses of 75 mg BID were well tolerated in healthy young subjects (n = 12). No MTD was determined in either study (Lucas et al., 1993).

The safety and tolerability of xanomeline was also evaluated in four panels of healthy elderly subjects (n = 16). Patients received one of four dose regimens of xanomeline: titration from 50 to 75 mg BID, titration from 15 to 25 mg TID, titration from 40 to 50 mg TID, or 40 mg TID. Adverse events such as moderate diarrhea, nausea, vomiting, diaphoresis, and hypotension were observed at all doses. One patient experienced moderate nausea and symptomatic hypotension at 50 mg TID, and no further doses were tested. The 50 mg TID dose was designated the MTD in this population.

Our double-blind, placebo-controlled, inpatient bridging study (Sramek et al., 1995c) was designed to evaluate the safety and tolerability of xanomeline in 48 patients with AD (20 males, 28 females; mean age 72 years). All patients met NINCDS-ADRDA and DSM-III-R criteria for AD, and scored four or less on the Modified Hachinski Ischemia Scale and between 10 and 26 on the MMSE at screening. None of the patients had a clinically significant condition that could interfere with study assessments.

The study was conducted in eight panels of six patients each. Patients were randomized to receive placebo (n = 2 per panel) or one of eight ascending fixed doses of xanomeline (n = 4 per panel) for seven days. Doses were 25, 35, 50, 60, 75, 90, 100, and 115 mg TID; progression to the next panel was contingent upon the tolerability of the previous panel.

One patient in each of the 60, 75, and 100 mg TID panels prematurely discontinued due to severe gastrointestinal adverse events. An additional patient receiving 100 mg TID elected to discontinue treatment on the first day of dosing due to adverse events that were considered moderate but tolerable by the investigator. The most common adverse events in patients receiving xanomeline were gastrointestinal disturbances (diarrhea, nausea, and abdominal pain), diaphoresis, lacrimation, and dizziness. In the 115 mg TID panel, one patient withdrew from the study after experiencing severe nausea and vomiting on the first day of dosing. The study was terminated when another patient in the 115 mg TID panel experienced severe hypotension, nausea, vomiting, diaphoresis, and pallor, as well as moderate tightness of the chest, hypersalivation, and lethargy. Thus, 115 mg TID was designated the MID and 100 mg TID was defined as the MTD of xanomeline in this population.

Although this bridging study was conducted in a relatively small number of patients, the results were highly predictive of the adverse event profile in a subsequent Phase II multicenter study. As seen in Table 5.4, the occurrence rates of the most common adverse events were very comparable between the two studies. This potential to identify adverse events of concern provides a means of establishing safety guidelines for higher dose ranges, and could improve the safety of Phase II trials. The MTD of 100 mg TID is twice the MTD reported for the healthy elderly population. This study directly illustrates the advantages of conducting a bridging study prior to dose selection for Phase II/III efficacy studies; in a recent efficacy study of xanomeline, only the highest (75 mg TID) of three doses evaluated (25,

Table 5.4 Incidence of adverse events: bridging study versus a large, multicenter study

Adverse Event	Bridging Study (n = 32)	Multicenter Study (n = 256)
Sweating	44%	46%
Nausea	38%	38%
Vomiting	25%	32%
Dyspepsia	22%	25%
Chills	25%	24%
Salivation	13%	11%
Chest Pain	6%	11%

50, and 75 mg TID) was found to be superior to placebo (Bodick et al., 1997). This dose would not have been included without the bridging study.

Lu 25-109

Lu 25-109 is a functionally selective partial M_1 agonist with M_2/M_3 antagonist properties which has demonstrated efficacy in preclinical cognitive test systems. In previous studies in healthy young and elderly male subjects, doses up to 30 mg were well tolerated. Common adverse events included headache, fatigue, diarrhea, and nausea. Most adverse events were mild in intensity, independent of dose, and short in duration. A separate double-blind, placebo-controlled, single- and multiple-dose study of Lu 25-109 in healthy elderly subjects reported that doses up to 130 mg QID were generally well tolerated. Although headache and dizziness were observed at all dose levels, most adverse events in this study were transient and mild in intensity.

Our double-blind, placebo-controlled, two-phase, inpatient bridging study assessed the safety and tolerability of Lu 25-109 in consecutive panels of AD patients (n = 32, 16 males, 16 females, mean age 69 years). Patients were required to meet NINCDS-ADRDA and DSM-IV criteria for probable AD, and to score between 10 and 26 on the MMSE and four or less on the Modified Hachinski Ischemia Scale. Patients were also required to be in good physical health, with no clinically significant conditions that could interfere with study assessments.

Phase I of the study was designed to determine the fixed-dose MTD of Lu 25-109 in five consecutive panels of 6 patients each (four Lu 25-109 and two placebo). Doses were originally set at 100,150, 200, 250, and 325 mg TID for seven days. Progression to the next panel was contingent upon the tolerability of the previous panel. In the first panel (100 mg TID), all four patients receiving Lu 25-109 experienced mild to moderate dizziness and nausea, and two of these patients reported mild to moderate increased salivation, flushing, and/or increased sweating. Due to the incidence of these adverse events, the scheduled doses for the Panels 2–5 were reduced to 125, 150, 200, and 225 mg TID, respectively. Cholinergic adverse events such as increased salivation, dizziness, gastrointestinal symptoms were observed at doses of 125–200 mg TID. One patient receiving 125 mg TID voluntarily withdrew from the study due to a condition unrelated to Lu 25-109, and another patient receiving 200 mg TID voluntarily withdrew due to moderate agitation and increased salivation. A final patient discontinued at 200 mg TID due to moderate to severe epigastric pain, vomiting, and intermittent dizziness. The 200 mg TID panel was terminated shortly thereafter, and the last panel was not conducted. Thus, the fixed-dose MID of Lu 25-109 was defined as 200 mg TID and the fixed-dose MTD was defined as 150 mg TID.

The second phase of the study was designed to determine if titration could improve the tolerability of Lu 25-109. A single panel of patients (six Lu 25-109 and two placebo) received doses that were 50%, 75%, 100%, 125%, and 150% of the fixed-dose MTD, with dose increases every four days. Thus, the dose schedule for Lu 25-109 was 75, 100, 150, 200, and 250 mg TID. Doses of 75 mg TID were well tolerated; mild dizziness and increased salivation were the only adverse events reported. However, the incidence and severity of adverse events increased with increasing dose. One patient experienced moderate abdominal pain, increased salivation, and dizziness at 200 mg TID, and was discontinued from the study. As titration did not appear to improve the tolerability of Lu 25-109, the panel was terminated. Thus, titration every four days did not appear to improve the tolerability of this compound.

In all of the above bridging studies, the difference in drug tolerance between AD patients and healthy subjects has several possible explanations. For example, the initial Phase I assessments in normal cohorts could be inaccurate, or the pharmacological changes associated with AD could account for the differences in drug response. Although the underlying mechanism is not known, the observed differences between patients and normals support the need for bridging studies prior to dose selection for Phase II/III.

EXAMPLE OF A BRIDGING STUDY IN ANXIETY

We recently conducted a bridging study of a novel potential anxiolytic, lesopitron, in patients with generalized anxiety disorder. This study employed the same design that we developed for trials of AD compounds, and illustrates the utility of bridging in multiple CNS indications.

Lesopitron

Lesopitron is a novel $5\text{-}HT_{1A}$ agonist chemically related to the azapirone class (Haj-Dahmane et al., 1994). In preclinical models of anxiety, lesopitron was equally effective or superior to diazepam and other azapirones with no apparent withdrawal symptoms (Costall et al., 1992; Barnes et al., 1992; Farre, 1992). Single, oral doses of lesopitron of 0.2 to 50 mg were well tolerated in healthy volunteers. A multiple-dose study of lesopitron in 60 healthy subjects found that doses up to 45 mg/day were well tolerated with no apparent relationship between dose and adverse events. Thus, 45 mg was designated the MTD in healthy subjects (data on file, Labratorios Dr. Esteve, S.A., Barcelona, Spain).

Our double-blind, placebo-controlled, inpatient bridging study (Sramek et al., 1996a) was conducted in 42 patients (27 males, 15 females; age range 20–61 years), divided into seven panels of six patients each. In each panel, four patients were randomized to receive lesopitron and two patients were randomized to receive placebo for 6.5 days. All patients had a primary diagnosis of GAD according to DSM-III-R criteria, modified to allow a minimum duration of anxiety symptoms of one month, and a Hamilton Rating Scale for Anxiety (HAM-A) score of at least 18 with a score greater than 2 on the 'anxious mood' item. Patients were also required to score no more than 16 on the 17-item Hamilton Rating Scale for Depression (HAM-D). Patients were excluded if their HAM-A score decreased by 25% or more between the screening and baseline assessments, if they had more than four panic attacks in the four weeks before screening, or if they had any clinically significant medical, neurological, or psychiatric disorders which could interfere with study evaluations.

Seven consecutive panels of patients were randomized to receive placebo or lesopitron at doses of 20, 25, 30, 40, 45, 50, and 60 mg BID. Progression to the next dose level was contingent upon the safety and tolerability of previous panels. Doses of 20–50 mg BID were well tolerated, with patients experiencing mild to moderate adverse events such as headache, dizziness, and nausea. At 60 mg BID, one patient experienced a severe episode of orthostatic hypotension accompanied by symptoms such as dizziness, lightheadedness, and diaphoresis. These symptoms resolved within one hour, and the patient completed the study. Two additional patients receiving lesopitron 60 mg BID experienced moderate to severe adverse events, including dizziness, lightheadedness, nausea, and headache. Due to the severity of these adverse events in half of the patients receiving lesopitron in this panel, 60 mg BID was designated the MID and 50 mg BID was designated the MTD. Thus, the MTD of lesopitron in patients with GAD was twice the highest dose tested in healthy volunteers, permitting the use of a higher dose range for Phase II efficacy trials.

There is some evidence that a bridging study might have been beneficial in the development of buspirone, another anxiolytic compound. Early studies of this compound evaluated what are now considered to be low doses, increasing only gradually to a maximum of 30 mg/day. These low doses are potentially responsible for the lack of positive findings in 9 of 11 pivotal efficacy studies (Psychopharmacologic Drugs Advisory Committee, 1983). Currently, the recommended dose of buspirone extends as high as 45–60 mg/day (Physician's Desk Reference, 1997). Thus, bridging studies could constitute an important new step in the development of compounds for the treatment of anxiety.

EXAMPLE OF A BRIDGING STUDY IN DEPRESSION

We also conducted a bridging study for the novel antidepressant ABT-200. As an MTD was not determined in the patient population prior to a preliminary Phase II study which indicated marginal efficacy, our bridging study was conducted in order to ensure that all safe and potentially therapeutic doses would be evaluated.

ABT-200

ABT-200 is a novel potential antidepressant and racemic mixture of two enantiomers. The SS enantiomer antagonizes the presynaptic uptake of norepinephrine, while the RR enantiomer antagonizes inhibitory α_2 autoreceptors (Zelle et al., 1994; Hancock et al., 1995). It has been hypothesized that these dual effects will result in a more rapid onset of antidepressant response (Johnson et al., 1980; Scott and Crews, 1983; Goldstein et al., 1985). In a previous pilot study of ABT-200 in patients with depression, no significant differences were found between 140 mg/day

ABT-200 and placebo for HAM-D total scores or CGI scores (Sramek et al., 1994/1995). However, core depression item scores on the HAM-D were significantly reduced in patients receiving ABT-200, suggesting the potential for therapeutic efficacy.

Our double-blind, placebo-controlled, outpatient bridging study was conducted in 12 depressed patients. Patients were required to meet DSM-III-R criteria for major depressive disorder with or without melancholia, to have a total score of at least 20 on the 24-item HAM-D, and a score of at least 2 on item 1 of the HAM-D. Patients were also required to have a HAM-A total score less than their HAM-D total score, a score of at least 8 on the Raskin Depression Scale, and a Covi-Anxiety Scale score less than their Raskin Depression Scale score. Exclusion criteria included clinically significant medical, neurological, or psychiatric disorders; a risk of suicide; ECT within six months of screening; psychiatric/psychological therapy within one month of screening; treatment with MAOIs or fluoxetine within four weeks of study treatment or any other antidepressants within two weeks of study treatment; or benzodiazepines (used for daytime sedation) within three weeks of study treatment.

The study was conducted in two panels. In the first panel, patients received placebo or were titrated over a three week period from an initial dose of 160 mg/day to a maximum maintenance dose of 240 mg/day ABT-200. In the second panel, patients received placebo or were titrated over a three week period from an initial dose of 160 mg/day to a maximum maintenance dose of 280 mg/day. Patients were to be maintained on their maximum maintenance dose for a total of four weeks.

All doses evaluated in this study were tolerated. The most common adverse events included lightheadedness, dizziness, headache, insomnia, drowsiness/sedation, and nausea. A total of three patients prematurely discontinued from the study due to adverse events: one due to lightheadedness, one due to decreased concentration and dizziness, and one due to nausea, dry mouth, and dizziness. Thus, this bridging study extended the usable dose range by 100% over doses that were previously not found to be efficacious in patients with depression.

Bridging Study of a Novel Antidepressant

In a proposed bridging study of a novel antidepressant compound, we developed a strategy to determine a tailored titration schedule based on the results of a previous fixed-dose study. Briefly, the occurrence rates of adverse events from a previous study evaluating five fixed doses of the compound were evaluated (by week) in order to determine the development of tolerance. For example, headache occurred in 4–6% of patients at each dose level, and evidence of tolerance was observed after approximately one week. Nausea occurred in 3–30% of patients, with tolerance developing in 8–10 days. In contrast, the incidence of dizziness ranged from 4–20%, increasing with dose, and required 1–3 weeks for tolerance to develop. Based on the profile of these adverse events, it appeared that at least one week was required to achieve tolerance for headache and nausea, and several weeks for dizziness. The incidence of other adverse events such as somnolence and insomnia were too low to evaluate tolerance over time.

Thus, a slow titration schedule for this compound over the first week of dosing is likely to decrease the incidence of dose-limiting adverse events such as headache and nausea, while titration over the first 2–3 weeks could help to decrease the incidence of dizziness. By examining the results of available fixed-dose studies, titration schedules tailored to the adverse event profile of the compound can be determined and tested, and higher doses can potentially be reached.

EXAMPLES OF BRIDGING STUDIES IN SCHIZOPHRENIA

Through our experience with bridging studies in schizophrenia, we have noted that compounds which require titration have a dose range that is less well defined, and may require a different study design. Many CNS compounds, antipsychotics in particular, require titration due to their adverse event profiles. For example, compounds such as clozapine and sertindole are α-adrenergic receptor antagonists, resulting in a high propensity for hypotension. There is evidence that adverse events such as hypotension can sometimes be ameliorated with titration. For example, in a study of the novel antipsychotic compound mazapertine (Kleinbloesem et al., 1996), tolerance to hypotension was induced with titration of the compound. Unfortunately, the need for titration can also slow the onset of antipsychotic effects if too much time is wasted before reaching a therapeutic dose. Thus, there is a need to determine not only an optimal dose range, but a rapid titration schedule to reach these doses quickly and safely.

A bridging study for a compound which needs to be titrated is typically divided into three distinct periods, each with a different objective (Sramek et al., 1997). As in the fixed-dose panel design, progression to the next phase is dependent upon the tolerability of the previous one. In Period I, the

MTD is determined in a panel of approximately eight patients on a slow titration schedule. The dosage is titrated upwards every three or more days (depending on the profile of the particular compound). The MTD from this period will serve as the maximum dose for subsequent panels. The maximum dose is sometimes also based on the NOAEL determined from preclinical studies in two species, even if an MTD is not reached in patients. If all doses in the first period are well tolerated, then an additional panel reaching higher doses may be required to define the MTD.

In Period II, the safety and tolerability of fixed doses of the study drug are evaluated in consecutive panels of up to eight patients each, until a fixed-dose MTD is reached. The doses tested are selected based on the slow titration MTD (e.g. 20%, 40%, 60%, 80%, and 100% of the slow-titration MTD). The fixed-dose MTD can then be used as the starting dose for subsequent titration panels. As it is generally beneficial to reach a target dose quickly, particularly for patients with acute symptoms, the identification of a higher initial dose could help to speed the titration process. Once the fixed-dose MTD is determined, Period III can evaluate a series of progressively faster titration schedules, beginning each panel with the fixed-dose MTD and ending with the slow titration MTD.

An added advantage of the three-period design is that a pharmaco-kinetic profile of the compound can be assessed in patients. Trough or peak concentrations approximating steady-state (depending on the half-life of the compound) can be drawn at the end of each dosing interval in the slow titration period (Period I), a full pharmacokinetic profile can be taken at several steady-state dose levels in the fixed-dose period (Period II), and the profile can also be repeated at the MTD dose in Period III, with an appropriate extension of the dosing at the conclusion of a rapid titration schedule. This extension of dosing also confirms that the MTD will be well tolerated after the dose is fully allowed to reach steady-state concentrations. In the event that the dosing of a particular antipsychotic compound does not require titration, panels of patients can still be used to evaluate the safety and tolerability of a series of fixed doses. As with the titration study, each of the consecutive panels is dependent on the tolerability of the previous dose level. It is still of some benefit to conclude the study with titration of the last panel, in order to determine any differences in tolerability between fixed and titrated doses, as titration may re-define the MTD. Bridging studies can thus determine the optimal dose range for Phase II studies in patients, and identify the best titration schedule to reach the top dose quickly.

We have recently conducted bridging studies of several novel antipsychotic compounds. Our results demonstrated that differences in tolerability between patients and healthy subjects necessitate dose-finding in patients prior to selecting a dose range for Phase II efficacy studies. Additionally, we will review our study evaluating the safety and tolerability of two rapid dose titration schedules of the antipsychotic sertindole. Finally, we will discuss our bioequivalence study of clozapine, and the safety reasons for conducting such trials in patients rather than normal volunteers.

MDL 100,907

MDL 100,907 is a potent and selective 5-HT$_{2A}$ antagonist which has demonstrated activity consistent with antipsychotic efficacy in animal models (Padich et al., 1996). In radioligand studies, MDL 100,907 demonstrated a pharmacological profile consistent with a low liability for EPS, and potential efficacy against negative symptoms (Kehne et al., 1996). Doses up to 72 mg were well tolerated in healthy subjects; however dose-limiting adverse events such as moderate to severe hypotension were observed at 138 mg.

We conducted a single-center, open-label bridging study to evaluate the safety and tolerability of single daily doses of MDL 100,907 in schizophrenic patients and to determine the MTD in this population. Thirty patients participated in this study in five consecutive panels of six patients each. Patients were required to meet DSM-IV criteria for primary Schizophrenia including presence of characteristic symptoms (excluding Schizoaffective and Mood Disorder with psychotic features), with an absence of any organic factor accounting for the symptomatology. They had no significant medical, neurological, or psychiatric disease, or any conditions which could potentially interfere with study evaluations. Patients could not have received fluphenazine injections within three weeks, haloperidol injections within six weeks, or an MAO inhibitor within one week prior to the washout phase; or fluoxetine within 30 days prior to the beginning of the study.

Following a three-day single-blind placebo washout period, patients received single daily fixed doses of MDL 100,907 for a total of seven days. Doses originally scheduled for the five panels were 20, 40, 80, 100, and 125 mg/day. In the first panel of patients, 20 mg MDL 100,907 was well tolerated, with only mild adverse events reported. Doses of 40 mg/day were also well tolerated; all adverse events were mild in intensity. The most common adverse events at these doses were lightheadedness and drowsiness.

At 80 mg/day, four of six patients experienced moderate lightheaded-ness approximately 2 h after the first dose of MDL 100,907. Three of these patients were no longer symptomatic after the second dose, and the fourth after the third dose, suggesting that tolerance to this adverse event developed rapidly. Only one other moderate adverse event (vomiting) was reported at this dose. However, due to these adverse events, the dose for the next panel was reduced to 60 mg.

The 60 mg/day dose of MDL 100,907 was well tolerated. Only one patient experienced a moderate adverse event (headache) judged to be related the study compound. The most common adverse events were drow-siness, insomnia, and headache. Based on the tolerability of this panel, and the possibility that divided doses would improve the tolerability of MDL 100,907, the dose for the last panel was set at 100 mg/day, administered BID for the first three days of treatment, and once daily (QD) for the remaining days. On this regimen, MDL 100,907 was well tolerated. Only one patient experienced a moderate adverse event (headache). The most common adverse events in this panel were drowsiness and headache. No severe or serious adverse events or EPS were observed in any study panel. Thus, the tolerability of higher doses of MDL 100,907 appears to be improved with divided dosing.

This bridging study demonstrated that single daily doses of MDL 100,907 were well tolerated up to 60 mg, and divided doses were well tolerated up to 100 mg. No MTD was determined; however, this study extended the usable dose range beyond the MTD in healthy volunteers (72 mg).

Iloperidone

Iloperidone is an atypical antipsychotic compound demonstrating affinity for D_2, D_3, D_4, $5-HT_{2A}$, $5-HT_6$, and $5-HT_7$ receptors with antagonistic action at α_1 adrenergic receptors (Kongsamut et al., 1996). In preclinical studies, iloperidone demonstrated efficacy in behavioral models predictive of antipsychotic activity against positive and negative symptoms (Corbett et al., 1993; Strupczewski et al., 1995), with a reduced liability for EPS (Szewczak et al., 1995). However, the α_1-adrenergic antagonist activity of iloperidone suggests a potential for orthostatic hypotension (Schwartz and Brotman, 1992). In a study in conscious dogs, iloperidone induced hypotension and peripheral vasodilation following doses of 1 and 10 mg/kg. In a design incorporating a three-day pre-treatment, however, only two of four dogs demonstrated hypotension and vasodilation (data on file, Hoechst Marion Roussel), suggesting that iloperidone's potential for orthostatic hypotension might be attenuated through dose titration.

In a single-dose safety and tolerability study of iloperidone in healthy, fasted subjects (n = 18), dose-limiting adverse events of orthostatic hypotension and dizziness were observed following iloperidone doses of 3 mg or greater (data on file, Hoechst Marion Roussel). In another study, fasted schizophrenic patients (n = 15) tolerated iloperidone titrated from 1– 8 mg/day over 22 days without any significant adverse events (data on file, Hoechst Marion Roussel).

We conducted a single-center, four-period (I–IV) bridging study to determine the safety and tolerability of single daily doses of iloperidone in schizophrenic patients. Twenty-four stable schizophrenic outpatients (mean age 37 years) participated in this inpatient study. Patients met DSM-IV criteria for Schizophrenia including presence of characteristic symptoms (excluding Schizoaffective Disorder and Mood Disorder with psychotic features), with an absence of any organic factor accounting for the symptomatology. They had no clinically significant medical, neurological, or psychiatric disease, or other abnormalities that could interfere with safety evaluations. Patients were also required to be daily cigarette smokers, in order to reduce potential pharmacokinetic variance caused by nicotine-induced stimulation of the hepatic metabolism of iloperidone. Due to a report of tinnitus in one patient in an earlier study, all patients were required to have a screening audiogram within normal limits for their age.

Study Period I was designed to determine the slow (every three days) titration MTD of iloperidone in a single panel of schizophrenic patients (n = 8). Following a four-day single-blind placebo washout period (Days -4 to-1), patients received an initial dose of iloperidone 2 mg/day for two days followed by three days each at 4, 6, 8, 12, 16, 20, 24, 28, and 32 mg. On this schedule, once-daily doses of iloperidone were well tolerated through the protocol maximum of 32 mg. One patient was discontinued from the study after experiencing a brief (1–2 s) syncopal episode approximately 2 h after receiving the initial dose of 2 mg iloperidone. The syncopal episode was judged to most likely be a first dose phenomenon, and we thus felt that continuation of the panel would not put other patients at risk. Due to this adverse event, however, 1 mg was defined as the initial dose for Study Periods III and IV. An additional patient in Study Period I was discontinued at 8 mg on Study Day 10 due to emerging psychosis. The most common adverse events were mild rhinitis and insomnia; moderate adverse events included fatigue and one episode of chest pain which was thoroughly evaluated and judged by a physician to be non-cardiac related.

Because an MTD was not reached, a decision was made to limit the top dose for subsequent periods to 24 mg.

Study Period II was originally designed to determine the fixed dose MTD, which would serve as the maximum initial dose of iloperidone for subsequent study periods. However, as an initial dose (1 mg) was selected in Study Period I, Study Period II was canceled.

In Study Period III, the tolerability of a more rapid (every two days) titration schedule was evaluated in a single panel of schizophrenic patients (n = 8). Doses were titrated from an initial dose of 1 mg to 2, 4, 8, 12, 16, 20, and 24 mg, with dose increases every two days. The rapid (every two day) titration of iloperidone was well tolerated for doses up to the maximum of 24 mg. One patient was discontinued at 16 mg on Day 12 due to emerging psychosis of moderate intensity. Other moderate adverse events included agitation, headache, and insomnia.

In Study Period IV, we evaluated the tolerability of a daily titration schedule in a single panel of schizophrenic patients (n = 8). Doses were identical to those in Study Period III, but dose escalation occurred every day. The daily titration of iloperidone was well tolerated for doses up to the maximum of 24 mg. Two patients discontinued at 24 mg on Days 9 and 11 due to emerging psychosis of moderate to severe intensity. Other moderate adverse events included fatigue, asthenia, dizziness, and insomnia.

The adverse events observed in this bridging study were similar in type and order of frequency to those in the Phase II efficacy study (n = 104) of iloperidone in patients with acute or relapsing schizophrenia (Borison et al., 1995). The four most common adverse events (rhinitis, insomnia, agitation, and headache) were identical for these two studies. Although the percentage of patients experiencing each adverse event was lower in the Phase II study, this difference is most likely due to the lower doses employed (2 and 4 mg BID). Thus, bridging studies can often be helpful in predicting prospective adverse events in subsequent, larger studies.

Although patients demonstrated reductions in supine to standing systolic and diastolic blood pressure in all study periods, this effect did not appear to be dose dependent, potentially due to development of tolerance with titration (Figure 5.3 a and b). Except for the patient with a brief syncopal episode shortly after receiving the higher initial dose of 2 mg, there were no other severe or serious adverse events judged to be related to study medication.

A total of four patients were discontinued from the study due to emerging psychosis. This study was conducted in stable schizophrenic outpatients who were voluntarily taken off their previous antipsychotic treatment regimen, and who might not have had sufficient time to respond

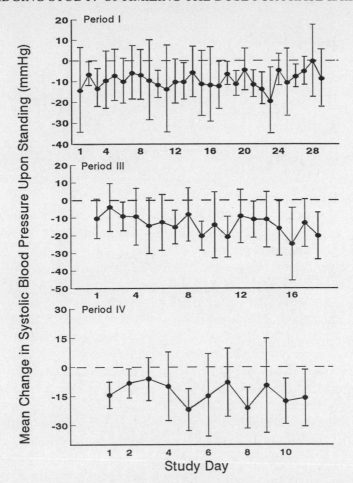

Figure 5.3 Mean change from baseline for orthostatic (a) systolic blood pressure in iloperidone-treated patients.

to the study drug before the end of the study. Thus, until further trials of a sufficient length are conducted, particularly in patients presenting with acute psychotic symptoms, no conclusions can be drawn regarding the efficacy of iloperidone. In a recent efficacy study of iloperidone in patients with acute or relapsing schizophrenia, 4 mg BID iloperidone was found to be superior to placebo in demonstrating improvement in mean PANSS total scores and CGI measures (Borison et al., 1995). Due to the deterioration and subsequent discontinuation of patients like those observed in this study, however, the size of the panels in bridging studies of antipsychotics are generally slightly larger than those for other indications.

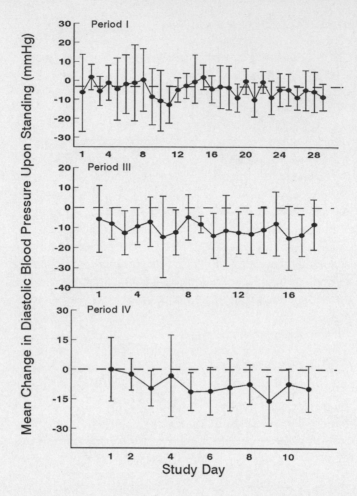

Figure 5.3 *(continued)* Mean change from baseline for orthostatic (b) diastolic blood pressure in iloperidone-treated patients. Reproduced by permission from Sramek et al., 1997.

In conclusion, this bridging study demonstrated that once daily doses up to at least 32 mg were tolerated on a slow titration schedule, and doses up to at least 24 mg were well tolerated on a rapid titration schedule (4 days to reach the reported threshold efficacy dose). Although no true MTD was determined, the doses tolerated by patients in the bridging study were ten times higher than single doses previously tolerated by healthy subjects and four times higher than the reported threshold dose for efficacy in a Phase II study of schizophrenic patients (Borison et al., 1995).

A Novel D_4/5-HT_2 Compound

We also conducted a bridging study of a novel compound which demonstrates potent activity at D_4 and 5-HT_{2A} receptors, with a low affinity for D_2 receptors. In preclinical studies, this compound demonstrated activity in several behavioral assays predictive of antipsychotic efficacy and did not cause catalepsy in mice at doses up to 160 mg/kg. In previous studies of healthy male volunteers, single doses of were tolerated up to 160 mg. At 300 mg, dose-limiting adverse events of hypotension and bradycardia were observed in four healthy subjects, potentially due to the drug's affinity for α_1-adrenergic receptors.

Our single-center, dose-rising, two-period bridging study was conducted in sequential panels of schizophrenic patients (n = 26). Subjects were male and female patients who met DSM-IV criteria for Schizophrenia with presence of characteristic symptoms (excluding Schizoaffective and Mood Disorder with psychotic features), with an absence of any known organic factors accounting for the symptomatology. They had no clinically significant medical, neurological, or psychiatric disease, or other abnormalities that could interfere with safety evaluations. Due to the potential hypotensive effects of this compound, all patients were required to have a supine and standing systolic blood pressure of ≥ 100 mg Hg, supine and standing diastolic blood pressure of ≥ 60 mm Hg, and a supine and standing pulse rate ≥ 50 bpm.

All patients completed a three-day single-blind placebo washout phase (Days -3 to -1) prior to receiving study medication. In the original study design, the objective of Study Period I was to determine the slow titration MTD of the compound in a single group of patients (n = 10), according to the schedule in Table 5.5.

On this slow titration schedule (increases of 100 mg every three days), the compound was well tolerated at doses up to 600 mg. Three patients were prematurely discontinued from the study. One patient withdrew at 300 mg due to an acute psychotic episode, another patient discontinued at 300 mg due to increased anxiety, and a third patient discontinued at 500 mg after experiencing a cardiac arrhythmia and a brief sinus pause of 1.44 seconds. This event was later judged to be not clinically significant by a cardiologist. The majority of other adverse events reported in Period I were considered to be mild in intensity; moderate adverse events included headache and anxiety. Although the 600 mg dose was well tolerated, no higher doses were tested due to findings which indicated that 600 mg is just below the preclinical NOAEL. Thus, no true MTD was reached in Period I.

Study Period II was designed to evaluate the tolerability of increasingly rapid titration schedules of this compound in four consecutive panels of schizophrenic patients (n = 6 per group):

Panel 1	100 → 600 mg over 8 days
Panel 2	100 → 600 mg over 6 days
Panel 3	100 → 600 mg over 4 days
Panel 4	600 mg on Day 1 (no titration)

Progression to each successive panel was only to be initiated if the previous panel was well tolerated. Panel 1 received an initial dose of 100 mg/day, followed by three days each at 200 and 400 mg. The final dose of 600 mg was maintained for three days. The compound was poorly tolerated on this titration schedule (increases of 200 mg every three days). One patient had a clinically significant elevation of liver enzymes at a dose of 400 mg and was withdrawn from the study. Two patients experienced moderate hypotension at 600 mg. One of these cases was accompanied by a brief syncopal episode, and the patient was discontinued from the study. Subsequently, all patients in Panel 1 were discontinued from the study for safety reasons.

As Panel 1 did not tolerate the compound well, the remaining panels were canceled, and an additional panel was included (Panel 2A) at an intermediate titration schedule (n = 10), shown in Table 5.6. Patients tolerated doses up to 600 mg on this titration schedule. One patient was prematurely discontinued from the study due to a moderate case of vertigo at 400 mg. Other moderate adverse events included insomnia, headache,

Table 5.5 Dosing schedule for Period 1

Day	Total Daily Dose of the D_4/5-HT_2 Compound	Administration
1	50 mg	50 mg QD
2–3	100 mg	50 mg BID
4–6	200 mg	100 mg BID
7–9	300 mg	150 mg BID
10–12	400 mg	200 mg BID
13–15	500 mg	250 mg BID
16–18	600 mg	300 mg BID

Table 5.6 An intermediate dose titration schedule

Day	Total Daily Dose of the D_4/5-HT_2 Compound	Administration
1	100 mg	50 mg BID
2–3	200 mg	100 mg BID
4–5	300 mg	150 mg BID
6–7	400 mg	200 mg BID
8–9	500 mg	250 mg BID
10–16	600 mg	300 mg BID

hypotension, hallucinations, increased salivation, and increased liver enzymes. The majority of adverse events for Panel 2A were considered to be mild. No serious adverse events or EPS were observed in any study period. Other than the elevation of liver enzymes in two patients, there were no clinically significant changes in laboratory measures.

Thus, this bridging study demonstrated that patients tolerated the compound at doses up to at least 600 mg on slow (increases of 100 mg every three days) and intermediate (increases of 100 mg every two days) titration schedules. Although this study did not find a true MTD, it did extend the usable dose range by almost 400%, and identified a safe and well-tolerated titration schedule for schizophrenic patients. A subsequent Phase II study of this compound did not find significant efficacy; however, this bridging study provides confidence that the clinically relevant dose range was thoroughly tested.

CI-1007

CI-1007 is a potent, orally active dopamine autoreceptor agonist and partial dopamine D_2/D_3 receptor agonist. In vivo, CI-1007 inhibits the firing of central dopaminergic neurons, and decreases the synthesis and release of dopamine in the brain. CI-1007 has also demonstrated antipsychotic-like activity with a reduced liability for EPS and tardive dyskinesia in preclinical models (Rugsley et al. 1995; Feng et al. 1997; Meltzer et al. 1995).

In a rising, single-dose tolerance study of CI-1007 in healthy subjects, oral doses of 5 mg were well tolerated. However, the incidence of adverse events, such as nausea, vomiting, and headache, increased at 10 mg and was dose-limiting at 15 mg. Orthostatic hypotension was also observed at 15 mg. Thus, 10 mg was designated the MTD in healthy subjects.

Our single-blind, rising, multiple-dose, inpatient bridging study (n = 16) was conducted in four consecutive panels of four patients each (Sramek et al., in press). Subjects were male and female schizophrenic patients who met DSM-IV criteria and required treatment with antipsychotic medication. They had no clinically significant medical, neurologic, or psychiatric disease, and no alcohol or drug abuse within six months prior to the study. Due to possible cardiovascular side effects with this autoreceptor agonist, patients were also required to have a standing (2 minute) systolic blood pressure > 100 mm Hg and heart rate < 100 bpm. Additionally, as the CYP2D6 locus is believed to be important for the drug metabolism of this compound, only patients with the normal/wild type CYP2D6 genotype were allowed to participate.

Following a four-day placebo washout period, patients were assigned to receive one of four doses of CI-1007 in Panel 1 (5 mg BID), Panel 2 (10 mg BID), Panel 3 (15 mg BID), or Panel 4 (20 mg BID). Patients in each panel received multiple doses of CI-1007 (administered every 12 hours) for four days, with a final dose on the morning of Day 5. Administration of higher doses of CI-1007 was contingent upon the tolerability of the lower doses.

CI-1007 was generally well tolerated over the dose range evaluated. The most common adverse events were nausea, vomiting, and headache, and were primarily mild in intensity. Adverse events were most commonly observed following the initial dose of CI-1007, and tended to decrease with repeated dosing.

The frequency and intensity of adverse events were greatest at the 20 mg BID dose level. Mild nausea (4 of 4 patients), moderate vomiting (3 of 4 patients), and transient symptomatic hypotension (systolic blood pressure 68–89 mmHg; 2 of 4 patients) were observed on the first three days of treatment at 20 mg BID. These symptoms lessened with subsequent doses, and CI-1007 was generally well tolerated for the remainder of the panel.

Modest reductions in blood pressure and increases in heart rate were observed in the majority of patients following the first few doses of CI-1007. One patient in Panel 3 experienced a brief (2–3 second), moderate syncopal episode following the initial 15 mg dose, but had no further complications for the remainder of the panel. No severe or serious adverse events or clinically significant abnormalities on physical exams, ECG, or laboratory tests were observed. No EPS was observed in any panel.

In conclusion, although no true MTD was determined, the results of this study indicate that schizophrenic patients tolerate higher initial doses of CI-1007 than healthy subjects.

Sertindole

In addition to the above bridging studies, we also conducted a study to evaluate the safety and tolerability of two rapid dose titration schedules of sertindole in patients with schizophrenia. This study demonstrates the utility of the bridging study not only in the initial stages of drug development, but also at the end of a development program. Sertindole is a potent $D_2/5-HT_2$ antagonist which has demonstrated efficacy in schizophrenic patients with an EPS profile indistinguishable from placebo (Zimbroff et al., 1997; van Kammen et al., 1996). However, the activity of sertindole at α_1-adrenergic receptors suggests a potential liability for orthostatic hypotension.

Sertindole has a well-defined therapeutic dose range, but requires titration up to an effective dose. A titration schedule with dose increases every three days was instituted for all sertindole studies after a Phase I study in which all five healthy subjects receiving single 8 mg doses of sertindole experienced tachycardia and associated clinically significant reductions in blood pressure, and three of the subjects experienced syncope. On this three-day titration schedule, orthostatic vital sign changes were reported in some patients, along with a 1–1.5% rate of syncope. However, overall results suggested that adaptation to the cardiovascular effects of sertindole may occur over time. In trials of healthy volunteers and schizophrenic patients prior to our study, sertindole was generally titrated at a rate of 4 mg every three days (Daniel et al., 1995).

Our open-label, multiple-dose study assessed the safety, tolerability, and pharmacokinetics of two rapid titration schedules of sertindole in schizophrenic patients. Sixteen patients (mean age 36 years) participated in the study in two sequential groups (n = 8 per group). Patients met DSM-IV criteria for primary Schizophrenia, and were free of any medical, neurological, or psychiatric conditions. All patients completed a four-day single-blind placebo washout before receiving sertindole on the first day of the study.

The first group of patients received sertindole, titrated from 4 to 24 mg in 4 mg increments with dose increases every two days. Overall, sertindole was well tolerated on this schedule. The most frequent adverse events were dry mouth, rhinitis, and headache. Only two patients experienced moderate adverse events (insomnia and myalgia).

In the second group, patients received the same doses as the previous group, but with dose increases every day. On this regimen, 88% of patients reported at least one moderate adverse event, including anxiety, asthenia, dizziness, insomnia, agitation, palpitations, headache, dry mouth, and vomiting. Mild to moderate tachycardia (heart rate $\geq$ 120 bpm and an increase of $\geq$ 20 upon orthostasis) was observed in all patients. Thus, the daily titration schedule was less well tolerated.

Overall, a titration rate of 4 mg every two days appear to be safe. The rate-limiting factor is tachycardia, although cases have been asymptomatic. Care must be taken before titrating sertindole every day; however, this titration schedule might be used if carefully monitored on an inpatient basis. The ability to safely titrate sertindole every other day potentially allows a 24 mg/day dose to be reached in 11 days, versus 16 days with three-day titration. Whether this time savings translates into a faster onset of treatment response will require further study.

Alternative Titration Strategies

The regimens proposed above for rapid titration panels are excellent general schemes which can be employed to reach the top dose as quickly as possible. However, there are occasions where a tailored bridging study can be employed latter in a compound's development in order to minimize adverse events which may prove to be excessive when the compound has not benefited from a bridging study early in its development. In such cases, it is very helpful to fine tune the titration by careful study of the time course of adverse events in Phase II studies.

For example, we examined the data from a number of Phase II trials of a $5HT_{1A}$ partial agonist in order to propose a titration rate which would allow for development of tolerance to serotonergic adverse events which were troublesome in clinical trials. By looking at the time course of adverse events over time and setting some parameters with which to characterize the data, one can get a handle on the time course needed for the development of tolerance. In these studies, the compound was administered on a fixed-dose regimen, in doses of 0.25, 1, 2, 3, or 4 mg per day. The parameters we chose to characterize the data were simple:

1. How many days of treatment did it take before a specific adverse event diminished greatly in frequency (drop of more than 75%), and
2. What was the percent mean incidence of these adverse events after three days of treatment? Thus characterized, we found the results listed in Table 5.7.

Thus, it becomes apparent that it will take up to several weeks to develop tolerance to a fixed dose of this compound, slightly longer for dizziness

Table 5.7 Mean incidence of adverse events (%) after three days of treatment

Adverse event	Dose				
	0.25 mg	1 mg	2 mg	3 mg	4 mg
Dizziness					
(days to tolerance)	7	14	18	20	20
(% after 3 days)	4	12	18	18	20
Nausea					
(days to tolerance)	10	8	9	9	14
(% after 3 days)	3	8	25	10	30

than for nausea. If higher doses are to be used (i.e., 2–4 mg), then it is also apparent that the incidence is related to the dose. One might then design a titration bridging study to go slowly up to the 2 mg dose in order to avoid these troublesome adverse events that often cause patients to discontinue treatment. However, after attaining 2 mg one might expect that the receptor dynamics will come into play and that tolerance will have developed such that further dose increases will be better tolerated. The compound should be titrated slowly from 0.25 mg per day up to 2 mg over the first two weeks of treatment (in this example, the condition to be treated is depression), and then when 2 mg is attained, we would predict that the incidence of adverse events will be much less, probably comparable to the lowest dose range of the compound. By utilizing titration, however, we might also expect that tolerance could be achieved in less than two weeks.

Therefore, after confirming the tolerance of the proposed titration scheme in a panel of patients, a second panel would be conducted to test the tolerability of a faster titration rate. A faster rate might allow tolerance to develop in one week instead of two, gaining valuable time in achieving a therapeutic dose in depressed patients and shortening the time to antidepressant response.

A Bioequivalence Study of Clozapine

As our bridging studies in schizophrenia have illustrated, patients can tolerate much higher doses of antipsychotics than healthy subjects. However, this difference appears to be even more pronounced for clozapine. While cardiac arrest has been reported in healthy male subjects at 25 mg Clozaril® (Pokorny et al., 1994), patients have been treated clinically at doses up to 900 mg/day. Thus, our bioequivalence and bioavailability study was conducted only in schizophrenic patients.

This inpatient, randomized, three-way crossover study was conducted in thirty stable schizophrenic patients between the ages of 18 and 55 years in three sequential cohorts. Patients were required to have a primary diagnosis of Schizophrenia, chronic (all types), in a residual phase or in remission according to DSM-III-R criteria. Patients were also required to have a total PANSS score of 90 or less; a score of 14 points or less on the following 4 items of the PANSS: conceptual disorganization, suspiciousness/persecution, hallucinatory behavior, and unusual thought content; and a score of 4 or less on the excitement, disturbance of volition, uncooperativeness, and poor impulse control items of the PANSS.

Following a three-day washout period, patients received Clozaril®, titrated upward from 25 mg/day (12.5 mg bid) to 150 mg/day (75 mg bid) over five days.   Patients were then randomized to receive one of the six treatment sequences shown in Table 5.8.

Samples for trough clozapine plasma concentrations were taken on the last four days of each one-week treatment period (I, II, and III), just prior to administration of the morning dose. In addition, blood samples for the measurement of plasma clozapine concentrations and pharmacokinetic determinations were taken at 0.5, 1.0, 2.0, 2.5, 3.0, 4.0, 6.0, 9.0, and 12.0 hours after the morning dose on the last day in each period. On the last day of Period III, blood samples were collected at 0.5. 1.0, 1.5, 2.0, 2.5, 3.0, 4.0, 6.0, 9.0, 12.0, 24.0, 36.0, 48.0, and 72.0 hours after the final morning dose. The steady-state pharmacokinetic parameters evaluated on the last day of dosing in each period were peak plasma concentration (C_{max}), plasma concentration 12.0 hours after dosing (C_{12}), plasma concentration prior to

Table 5.8 Six different treatment sequences

Sequence	Titration Period (Days 1–5)	Period I (Days 6–12)	Period II (Days 13–19)	Period III (Days 20–26)
1	12.5 → 75 mg bid	A	B	C
2	12.5 → 75 mg bid	B	C	A
3	12.5 → 75 mg bid	C	A	B
4	12.5 → 75 mg bid	B	A	C
5	12.5 → 75 mg bid	A	C	B
6	12.5 → 75 mg bid	C	B	A

A = Clozaril® 100 mg tablets: one tablet BID.
B = Clozapine 25 mg tablets: four tablets BID.
C = Clozapine 100 mg tablets: one tablet BID.

dosing (C_0), time to peak plasma concentration (T_{max}), and area under the concentration-time curve (AUC_{0-12}).

Final evaluations were performed on Day 29, and providing there were no clinically significant conditions requiring further hospitalization, all patients were discharged. Prior to discharge, patients were restarted on their prior antipsychotic medication.

Thirty schizophrenic patients (22 males, 8 females; mean age 35 years) participated in this study. Three patients were discontinued from the study; one due to elevated liver enzymes and two due to withdrawal of consent. In the first cohort of patients (n = 10) six patients experienced clinically significant orthostatic blood pressure changes following the first 12.5 mg dose of clozapine. Five of the six patients experienced dizziness, lightheadedness, pallor, and diaphoresis, and one of these five patients experienced a syncopal episode. Five of the six cases resolved during the titration period; one patient continued to experience lightheadedness throughout the study. Due to these adverse events, a decision was made to hospitalize these patients, as well as subsequent cohorts, during the initial titration period and to closely monitor vital signs. There were no other clinically significant blood pressure changes during the study.

Both the 100 mg and 4 x 25 mg tablet strengths of the generic product clozapine (Creighton) were found to be bioequivalent to the Clozaril® 100 mg tablet (Sandoz). A summary of the pharmacokinetic results is shown in Table 5.9. Five of the 27 patients (18.5%) who completed the study were excluded from the statistical analysis because they did not meet the assumption of absence of differential status between study periods crucial to the study's crossover design. Two of these patients failed to achieve steady state conditions as evidenced by long clozapine half-lives (40.8 hours and 140.8 hours), two patients exhibited trough concentrations varying > 25 ng/ml/day, and one patient showed clinically significant increases in glucose, triglyceride, cholesterol, globulin, and total protein concentrations between Periods I and III.

As patients included in the study were not treatment-refractory, but stable outpatients who were receiving typical antipsychotics as maintenance treatment, it is possible that the high percentage of orthostatic hypotension observed in this study (20%), as compared to previous studies of clozapine (9%) (Physician's Desk Reference, 1997), is due to a greater susceptibility of this population to cardiovascular side effects than chronic, treatment refractory patients. Our study of this population may have clinical relevance, however, as clozapine treatment is increasingly broadened to schizophrenic patients who may have good clinical response to typical

Table 5.9 Pharmacokinetic Results

	Mean ± Standard Deviation (n = 22)			90% Confidence Intervals (and ratios)	
	1 x 100 mg Clozaril®	4 x 25 mg Clozapine	1 x 100 mg Clozapine	4 x 25 mg Clozapine vs. 1 x 100 mg Clozapine	1 x 100 mg Clozapine vs. 1 x 100 mg Clozaril®
AUC (ng·hr/ml)	2547 ± 1429	2683 ± 1613	2781 ± 1775	91–108 (99)	97–114 (105)
C_{max} (ng/ml)	317 ± 163	351 ±167	358 ± 184	92–112 (101)	102–125 (113)
C_0 (ng/ml)	149 ± 95	155 ± 106	160 ± 128	93–111 (102)	91–109 (100)
C_{12} (ng/ml)	141 ± 79	140 ± 106	153 ± 130	87–108 (97)	89–111 (99)
T_{max} (hr)	2.50 ± 1.09	2.02 ± 0.832	1.93 ± 0.758	-	-

neuroleptics but are hypersensitive to their adverse effects (Carpenter et al.,1995), or to patients with other psychiatric or neurological disorders (Ranjan and Meltzer, 1996; Calabrese et al., 1996; Oberholzer et al., 1992; Chacko et al., 1995).

Although there were no significant differences in safety between groups in this study, a high incidence (6 out of 30 patients, 20%) of orthostatic hypotension was found with the initial titration of Clozaril,® emphasizing the need for careful monitoring, even in the patient population.

PHARMACOKINETIC/PHARMACODYNAMIC ASSESSMENTS IN THE BRIDGING STUDY

The evaluation of pharmacokinetic/pharmacodynamic (PK/PD) relationships has increasingly been recognized as an important element of early drug development. Peck et al. (1994) noted that a failure to define a relationship between dose, concentration, and treatment response often leads to unacceptable toxicity or marginal evidence of efficacy due to inappropriate doses and a lack of information on how to individualize dosing in Phase III. Incorporation of PK/PD measures at a stage early enough to influence subsequent development, however, may assist in the identification of optimal dosing regimens, and could contribute to an acceleration of drug development. Furthermore, PK/PD measures can lead to an increased understanding of a drug's mechanism of action, as well as information that could be useful in drug labeling.

The importance of PK/PD studies has also been recognized from the regulatory perspective.   In this arena, PK/PD studies could provide flexibility in the regulatory review process (Lesko and Williams, 1994). For example, bioequivalence criteria might be relaxed based on a better understanding of PK/PD relationships, and the intra-individual variability of these relationships.   Optimizing dose regimens with PK/PD information could also reduce drug development costs by more efficiently fulfilling requirements for administration of investigational compound to patients at clinically effective doses.

The bridging study provides a unique opportunity to explore PK/PD relationships in the target patient population for a larger range of doses than those that will most likely be employed at later stages. The incorporation of PK/PD measures in the bridging study could assist in more completely characterizing the acute pharmacologic effects of the compound, and defining the relationship of these effects to both dose and the incidence of adverse events. Additionally, PK/PD models could be constructed for use in later phases to assist in the initiation and adjustment of dosing in individual patients.

One potential challenge in establishing a PK/PD relationship, however, is defining an appropriate pharmacodynamic endpoint. Potential pitfalls in selecting a pharmacodynamic endpoint include drug assay problems or lack of accessible biological samples, lack of an immediate pharmacologic effect that can be related to pharmacokinetic measures, or lack of a relationship between a quantifiable pharmacologic effect and long-term clinical benefit (Williams, 1992). In many CNS indications, the logical pharmacodynamic endpoint is a surrogate marker and not a therapeutic outcome measure. For example, a study of an antidepressant might assess serotonin metabolite levels, which, although an easily quantifiable measure, might not reveal relevant information about the quality of life of a patient with depression. Studies of compounds for AD also rely on surrogate pharmacodynamic endpoints, such as AChE inhibition. However, a PK/PD study employing surrogate endpoints can help to confirm a compound's mechanism of action, and can provide useful preliminary concentration-response information.

The Dynabridge Study

It is important to bear in mind that PK/PD relationships may differ between the central and peripheral compartments. For CNS compounds, the action of the drug in the central compartment is of primary interest, although a knowledge of peripheral PK/PD parameters may be helpful in understanding adverse events. Thus, the assumption that a peripheral measure is a good indicator of central pharmacokinetics or activities should be tested early in development. For example, the utility of peripheral AChE inhibition as a measure of central cholinesterase inhibition cannot be taken for granted. The half-life of erythrocyte AChE inhibition after dosing with the irreversible cholinesterase inhibitor, metrifonate, appears to depend on the rate of synthesis of new red blood cells. There is no reason to expect that this will have any relationship with the rate of recovery of central activity. Differences in selectivity between central and peripheral forms of an enzyme may also play a role, as in the case of SDZ ENA 713, which is specific for central AChE and inhibits peripheral AChE only minimally. On the other hand, verification that a peripheral marker does indeed correspond to central activity can greatly simplify the monitoring of patients.

To assess central PK/PD relationships and their connection to peripheral PK/PD parameters, we developed 'dynabridge' methodology. A *dynabridge study* is a PK/PD CSF study in the patient population. As the name suggests, dynabridge studies extend the bridging concept of early exploratory studies in the patient population. In a dynabridge study, the focus moves beyond dose-finding and safety/tolerance to pharmacodynamic indicators of drug activity. A distinguishing feature of these studies is continuous CSF sampling which allows the determination of central PK/PD time courses. CSF is analyzed for drug and metabolite concentrations, as well as for measures of drug activity (e.g., enzyme activities, neurotransmitter levels, etc.). Peripheral PK/PD parameters are monitored simultaneously. Potential correlations with psychiatric or neurologic rating scales and/or neuropsychological tests are also investigated. As a result of a dynabridge study, the time course of drug activity across the potential dosing range is determined, permitting optimal design of dosing prior to efficacy trials. In addition, the central activity of the compound is confirmed and potential surrogate markers are explored.

A Dynabridge Study of an Acetylcholinesterase Inhibitor

Recently, we conducted a dynabridge study of an acetylcholinesterase inhibitor in patients with probable AD. This single-center, open-label, multiple-dose study was designed to evaluate the effects of this compound on AChE and BChE activity in CSF, and to correlate these parameters with pharmacokinetic measures and cognitive performance on the Computerized Neuropsychological Test Battery (CNTB).   Eighteen patients (nine males, nine females; mean age 63 years) meeting NINCDS-ADRDA criteria for probable AD were enrolled in this study in six sequential groups of three patients each. Patients were required to score between 10 and 26 on the MMSE and no more than 4 on the Modified Hachinski Ischemia Scale. Patients were also required to be in good physical health, with no medical, neurological, or psychiatric conditions that could potentially alter the absorption, accumulation, metabolism, or excretion of any drug. Patients were excluded if they had received any psychoactive medication, including tranquilizers within two weeks, antidepressants within one month, or neuroleptics within two months.

Patients were admitted to the hospital for baseline assessments, and received the investigational compound, titrated from 1 mg BID to one of six target dose levels (1, 2, 3, 4, 5, or 6 mg BID) in 1 mg BID/week increments. Study medication was then administered on an outpatient basis, with patients returning to the hospital for weekly inpatient safety evaluations. Patients were readmitted to the hospital when they had tolerated their target dose for at least three days, and received a final dose of study medication on the following morning. In order to evaluate the cognitive effects of the compound, patients were administered the CNTB at screening (for practice), at baseline, and on the day prior to receiving the last dose of study medication.

A total of 7 ml of blood for the determination of plasma concentrations of the compound and its metabolite, was collected from each patient 30 minutes prior to and 0.5, 1, 1.5, 2, 3, 4, 6, 8, 10, 12, and 24 hours after administration of the final dose. A continuous CSF sampling procedure for the determination of study compound concentrations and AChE and BChE activity was also performed during the 30 minutes prior to and for 12 hours after the final dose. For this procedure, patients were placed on their sides and received a local anesthetic in the lumbar area. A needle containing a 19-gauge, sterile, flexible, epidural catheter was placed in the L2-3 or L3-4 interspace under fluoroscopy, using aseptic techniques. The needle was then removed while the catheter was threaded into the spinal fluid sac, and taped into place or secured with a suture. A peristaltic pump was used for continuous CSF collection, at a rate of 1.2 ml per 12 minutes.

Plasma and CSF concentrations of the compound and its metabolite were determined by a specific gas chromatography-mass spectrometry method, with electron impact ionization (sensitivity 0.2 ng/ml). The measurement of AChE and BChE enzyme activity in CSF and plasma was carried out according the method of Ellman et al (1961). Calculation of enzyme activity was based on a change in optical density in the linear range over time using the molecular extinction coefficient of the reaction product $(13.3 \text{ cm}^2/\mu\text{mole})$.

The investigational compound was rapidly absorbed and quickly eliminated following the administration of a single dose, with a half-life of 1.1 to1.6 hours over the 1–6 mg BID dose range. Its metabolite was rapidly formed in all patients, and plasma concentrations of the metabolite declined at a slower rate than the parent compound. Plasma concentrations of both the study compound and its metabolite tended to increase with dose; significant correlations were observed between dose and the AUC_{0-12} of the plasma concentration of the compound ($r = 0.84$, $p < 0.0001$) and its metabolite ($r = 0.93$, $p < 0.0001$). Dose was also significantly correlated with the C_{max} of the plasma concentration of the compound ($r = 0.87$, $p < 0.0001$) and its metabolite ($r = 0.89$, $p < 0.0001$).

A dose-concentration relationship was also observed for CSF pharmacokinetic measures. Significant correlations were found between dose and CSF AUC_{0-12} values for the study compound ($r = 0.84$, $p < 0.0001$) and its metabolite ($r = 0.92$, $p < 0.0001$), and between dose and the C_{max} of the study compound ($r = 0.86$, $p < 0.0001$) and its metabolite ($r = 0.89$, $p < 0.0001$). The half-life of the compound in CSF ranged from 0.31 to 3 hours.

Administration of the study compound resulted in dose-dependent inhibition of CSF AChE which reached significance ($p < 0.05$) for all dose levels except 1 mg BID. Maximum inhibition (61.7%) was observed in the 6 mg BID group at 5.6 hours post-dose, and recovered steadily over the remaining 6 hours. The relationship between the mean concentration of the compound in CSF and the mean percent change in CSF AChE activity following a dose of 6 mg BID is shown in Figure 5.4. Significant inhibition of CSF BChE activity was also observed for all dose levels except 2 mg BID. Maximum BChE inhibition was observed in the 3 mg BID group at 11.6 hours post-dose, but inhibition was variable over the time points evaluated for all dose levels. Although significant reductions of BChE activity were observed in plasma, inhibition was lower than for CSF at all dose levels. The time courses of plasma BChE inhibition, CSF AChE inhibition, and CSF BChE inhibition all differed from each other and from the time courses of the drug and its metabolite. Thus, plasma cholinesterase appears to have minimal utility as a surrogate marker for drug action.

Significant correlations were observed between improvement on the CNTB Summary Score from baseline to the post-dose evaluation and the AUC_{0-12} of AChE ($p < 0.05$) and BChE ($p < 0.01$) in CSF. The 6 mg BID treatment group also demonstrated significant improvement relative to

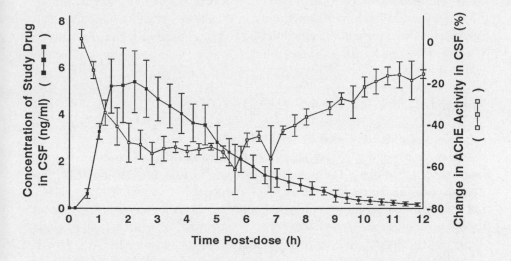

Figure 5.4 The time course of mean (± S.E.) study compound concentration in CSF and the mean (± S.E.) percent change in CSF AChE activity following a dose of 6 mg bid (n = 3).

baseline on the Paired Associate Learning With Selective Reminding (p = 0.02) and Paired Associate Learning/Delayed Recall (p = 0.04) subtests of the CNTB. In contrast to the CSF cholinesterases, plasma BChE inhibition did not appear to be correlated to neurophysiological measures.

Overall, the compound was well tolerated in this population over the dose range evaluated. The majority of adverse events, including headache, nausea, and dizziness, were rated as mild in intensity and were considered to be related to the lumbar catheterization procedures. No serious or severe adverse events, or clinically significant changes in vital signs, ECG, or clinical laboratory tests were reported.

This study illustrates the utility of assessing both central and peripheral pharmacokinetic parameters, as the half-life of the compound appears to be longer in CSF than in plasma. Additionally, the inclusion of PK/PD measures provides valuable information regarding adequate dosing intervals; the time course of AChE inhibition in CSF in this study justifies BID dosing with this compound. Thus, the compound produced a rapid, sustained, and dose-dependent inhibition of CSF AChE which was attended by cognitive enhancement. Although significant inhibition was also observed for BChE in plasma and CSF, the magnitude of inhibition was more variable, consistent with the selectivity of AChE as the principal target of this compound. The utility of measuring central cholinesterase inhibition rather than peripheral inhibition was also apparent. The results of this dynabridge study confirm the central action of this compound, and provide useful information on the PK/PD relationship for the dose range evaluated.

SPECIAL CONSIDERATIONS IN THE BRIDGING STUDY

The studies reviewed in this chapter illustrate the importance of bridging in optimizing dose selection for Phase II/III. However, certain aspects of the bridging study warrant further discussion. Because bridging studies explore the upper limits of a compound's tolerable dose range, patients are required to be in good physical health without concomitant medical conditions or medications. Patients are also under close supervision during the bridging study, which minimizes issues of compliance. Thus, we recommend that later efficacy trials be conducted using initial doses somewhat lower than the MTD, bearing in mind that the population in large outpatient studies will often display a greater inter-patient variability and will be less closely monitored.

Although the small panel sizes in a bridging study generally preclude formal statistical analysis, a bridging study does have the statistical power to reveal common, acute adverse events. If the probability of a given dose being toxic is 0.5, then the inclusion of at least four patients on active medication per panel allows us to be 94% confident that the dose is non-toxic (Geller, 1984). This confidence level is increased to 98% when six patients per panel on active compound are included. However, as the bridging study attempts to identify doses that are sub-toxic, the inclusion of a greater number of patients per panel is desirable. Thus, the data generated in a bridging study are sufficient to provide reliable information about the overall adverse event dose-response curve and to produce descriptive statistics. While long-term toxicity is not addressed by bridging studies, most acute effects should be accurately predicted. As illustrated by xanomeline, bridging studies have been shown to be highly predictive of the acute adverse event profiles found in Phase II, and thus are valuable in optimizing the safety of these trials.

Table 5.10 Types of studies conducted in the development of a new compound

Study Type	Population	Goal/Outcome
Single-dose escalation	Healthy volunteers	Safety/tolerance/pharmacokinetics
Multiple-dose escalation	Healthy volunteers	Safety/tolerance/pharmacokinetics
Food interaction	Healthy volunteers	Effect of food on pharmacokinetics
Bridging study	Patients	Safety/tolerance; MTD
Dynabridge study	Patients	Central PK/PD
Dose-ranging efficacy	Patients	Efficacy and long-term safety

CONCLUSIONS

Thus, there are several stages involved in the development of a potential new compound (Table 5.10). In our opinion, the studies listed in Table 5.10 are the core or critical studies that need to be conducted in order to make critical go/no-go decisions. Initial clinical development might proceed with placebo-controlled single dose escalation studies in healthy subjects, with a dose range based on preclinical data such as the NOAEL. Escalation to a range that allows adequate estimation of the compound's pharmacokinetics (particularly dose proportionality) and a definite adverse event profile is desirable at this stage. Following these studies, several multiple-dose panels in healthy subjects should be conducted in order to construct steady-state pharmacokinetic profiles, and to determine the linearity of the kinetics and additional safety data. A food interaction study should also be conducted at this time. These studies all lay the groundwork for the bridging and dynabridge studies, which will evaluate optimal dose parameters and schedules for studies in Phase II/III. In this way, bridging studies are central to the transition from studies in healthy subjects to dose-ranging and efficacy studies in patients. Of course, additional efficacy studies, some including active control arms, and clinical pharmacology studies (drug interactions, special populations or medical conditions) will be conducted later in development if efficacy is supported by earlier stages.

The examples reviewed in this chapter illustrate the importance of incorporating the target population into early drug development in order to optimize dose selection for Phase II/III. By providing information on differences in tolerance between healthy subjects and the target patient population, bridging and dynabridge studies constitute a vital contribution to the creation of an accelerated, rational drug development program.

REFERENCES

Anand R, Hartman R. Strategies for the optimal development of an anti-dementia drug. Presented at the *Fifth International Conference on Alzheimer's Disease and Related Disorders*, July 24–29, 1996; Osaka, Japan.

Barnes NM, Cheng CHK, Costall B, Ge J, Kelley ME, Naylor RJ. Profiles of interaction of R(+)/S(-)-zacopride and anxiolytic agents in a mouse model. *Eur J Pharmacol* 1992; **218**: 91–100.

Bodick NC, Offen WW, Levey AI, Cutler NR, Gauthier SG, Satlin A, Shannon HE, Tollefson GD, Rasmussen K, Bymaster FP, Hurley DJ, Potter WZ, Paul SM. Effects of xanomeline, a selective muscarinic receptor agonist, on cognitive function and behavioral symptoms in Alzheimer's disease. *Arch Neurol* 1997; **54**: 465–473.

Borison RL, Huff FJ, Varaklis J, Griffiths L, Ramaswamy R, Shipley JE. Efficacy of 2 and 4 mg bid iloperidone (HP 873) administered to schizophrenic patients for 42 days. Presented at the *34th Meeting of the American College of Neuropsychopharmacology*; San Juan, Puerto Rico, December 11–15, 1995; p. 135.

Calabrese JR, Kimmel SE, Woyshville MJ, Rapport DJ, et al. Clozapine for treatment-refractory mania. *Am J Psychiatry* 1996; **153**(6): 759–764.

Carpenter WT Jr, Conley RR, Buchanan RW, Breier A, Tamminga CA. Patient response resource management: another view of clozapine treatment in schizophrenia. *Am J Psychiatry* 1995; **152**(6): 827–832.

Chako RC, Hurley RA, Harper RG, Jankovic J, Cardoso F. Clozapine for acute and maintenance treatment of psychosis in Parkinson's disease. *J Neuropsychiatry Clin Neurosci* 1995; **7**(4): 471–475.

Costall B, Domeney AM, Kelly ME, Martinez L, Naylor RJ, Farre AJ. Profile of action of a novel 5-hydroxytryptamine$_{1A}$ receptor ligand E-4424 to inhibit aversive behavior in the mouse, rat, and marmoset. *J Pharmacol Exp Ther* 1992; **262**: 90–98.

Corbett R, Hartman H, Kerman LL, Woods AT, Strupczewski JT, Helsley GC, Conway PC, Dunn RW. Effects of atypical antipsychotic agents on social behavior in rodents. *Pharmacol Biochem Behav* 1993; **45**(1): 9–17.

Cutler NR, Murphy MF, Nash RJ, Prior PL, De Luna DM. Clinical safety, tolerance, and plasma levels of the oral anticholinesterase 1,2,3,4-tetrahydro-9-aminoacridin-1-oL-maleate (HP 029) in Alzheimer's disease: preliminary findings. *J Clin Pharmacol* 1990; **30**(6): 556–561.

Cutler NR, Sramek JJ. Scientific and ethical concerns in clinical trials in Alzheimer's patients: the bridging study. *Eur J Clin Pharmacol* 1995a; **48**: 421–428.

Cutler NR, Sramek JJ. The target population in phase I clinical trials of cholinergic compounds in Alzheimer's disease: the role of the 'bridging study.' *Alzheimer Dis Assoc Disord* 1995b; **9**:139–145.

Cutler NR, Sramek JJ, Kilborn JR. The bridging concept: optimizing the dose for phase II/III in Alzheimer's disease. *Neurodegeneration* 1996; **5**(4): 511–514.

Cutler NR, Sramek JJ, Murphy MF. The use of bridging studies in drug development for Alzheimer's disease therapeutics. In: Cutler NR, Gottfries CG, and Siegfried K eds. *Alzheimer's Disease: Clinical and Treatment Perspectives*. Chichester, England: John Wiley & Sons, 1995.

Cutler NR, Sramek JJ, Veroff AE. Alzheimer's disease: *Optimizing Drug Development Strategies*. Chichester, England: John Wiley & Sons, 1994.

Daniel D, Targum S, Zimbroff D, Mack R, Zborowski J, Morris D, Sebree T, Wallin B. Efficacy, safety, and dose response of three doses of sertindole and three doses of haldol in schizophrenic patients. Presented at the *34th Annual Meeting of the American College of Neuropsychopharmacology,* San Juan, Puerto Rico, Dec. 11–15, 1995.

Davis R, Raby C, Callahan MJ, Lipinski W, Schwarz R, Dudley DT, Lauffer D, Reece P, Jaen J, Tecle H. Subtype selective muscarinic agonists: potential therapeutic agents for Alzheimer's disease. *Prog Brain Res* 1993; **98**: 439–445.

Ellman GL, Courtney KD, Andres V, Featherstone RM. A new and rapid colorimetric determination of acetylcholinesterase activity. *Biochem Pharmacol* 1961; **7**: 88–95.

Enz A, Amsutz R, Boddeke H, Gmelin G, Malanowski J. Brain selective inhibition of acetylcholinesterase: a novel approach to therapy for Alzheimer's disease. *Prog Brain Res* 1993; **98**: 431–438.

Farde L, Sukara T, Halldin C. Radioligands for PET-examination of central muscarinic receptors. Presented at the *Alzheimer's and Parkinson's Diseases Recent Developments, Third International Conference*, Chicago, IL, November 1–6, 1993.

Farre AJ. CNS profile of lesopitron, a new 5-HT$_{1A}$ receptor ligand. *Behav Pharmacol* 1992; **3**(Suppl 1): 23.

Feng MR, Corbin AE, Wang Y, Christoffersen CL, Wiley JN, Strenkoski CA, Tucker EV, Ninteman FW, Meltzer LT, Heffner TG, Wright DS. Pharmacokinetics and pharmacodynamics of an investigational antipsychotic agent, CI-1007, in rats and monkeys. *Pharm Res* 1997; **14**(3): 329–336.

Geller NL. Design of phase I and II clinical trials in cancer: a statistician's view. *Cancer Invest* 1984; **2**: 483–491.

Goldberg MR, Barchowsky A, McCrea J, et al. Heptylphysostigmine (L-693,487): safety and cholinesterase inhibition in a placebo-controlled rising-dose healthy volunteers study. Presented at the *Second International Springfield Symposium on Advances in Alzheimer Therapy*, May, 1991.

Goldstein JM, Knobloch-Litwin LC, Malick JB. Behavioral evidence for beta-adrenoceptor subsensitivity after subacute antidepressant/alpha 2-adrenoceptor antagonist treatment. *Naunyn Schmiedebergs Arch Pharmacol* 1985; **329**(4): 355–358.

Grof P, Akhter MI, Campbell M. *Clinical Evaluation of Psychotropic Drugs for Psychiatric Disorders: Principles and Proposed Guidelines*. Seattle: Hogrefe & Huber, 1993.

Haj-Dahmane S, Jolas T, Laporte AM, Gozlan H, Farre AJ, Hamon M, Lanfumey L. Interactions of lesopitron (E-4424) with central 5-HT$_{1A}$ receptors: in vitro and in vivo studies in the rat. *Eur J Pharmacol* 1994; **255**: 185–196.

Hancock AA, Buckner SA, Giardina WJ, Brune ME, Lee JY, Morse PA, Oheim KW, Stanisic DS, Warner RW, Kerkman DJ, DeBernardis JF. Preclinical pharmacological actions of (±)-(1'R*, 3R*)-3-phenyl-1-[(1',2',3',4'-tetrahyrdro-5',6'-methylene-dioxy-1'-naphthalenyl methyl] pyrrolidine methanesulfonate (ABT-200), a potential antidepressant agent that antagonizes alpha-2 adrenergic receptors and inhibits the neuronal uptake of norepinephrine. *J Pharmacol Exp Ther* 1995; **272**: 1160–1167.

Hinz V, Grewig S, Schmidt BH. Metrifonate and dichlorvos: effects of a single oral administration on cholinesterase activity in rat brain and blood. *Neurochem Res* 1996; **21**(3): 339–345.

Itoh A, Nitta A, Hirose M, Hasegawa T, Nabeshima T. Effects of metrifonate on impairment of learning and dysfunction of cholinergic neuronal system in basal forebrain-lesioned rats. *Behav Brain Res* 1997a; **83**(1–2): 165–167.

Itoh A, Nitta A, Katono Y, Usui M, Naruhashi K, Iida R, Hasegawa T, Nabeshima T. Effects of metrifonate on memory impairment and cholinergic dysfunction in rats. *Eur J Pharmacol* 1997b; **322**(1): 11–19.

Jackson WJ, Buccafusco JJ, Terry AV, Turk DJ, Rush DK. Velnacrine maleate improves delayed matching performance by aged monkeys. *Psychopharmacology (Berl)* 1995; **119**(4): 391–398.

Johnson RW, Reisine T, Spotnitz S, Wiech N, Ursillo R, Yamamura HI. Effects of desipramine and yohimbine on alpha 2- and beta-adrenoreceptor sensitivity. *Eur J Pharmacol* 1980; **67**(1): 123–127.

Kehne JH, Baron BM, Carr AA, Chaney SF, Elands J, Feldman DJ, Frank RA, van Giersbergen PL, McClosky TC, Johnson MP, McCarty DR, Poirot M, Senyah Y, Siegel BW, Widmaier C. Preclinical characterization of the potential of the putative atypical antipsychotic MDL 100,907 as a potent 5-HT$_{2A}$ antagonist with a favorable CNS safety profile. *J Pharmacol Exp Ther* 1996; **277**(2): 968–981.

Kleinbloesem CH, Jaquet-Muller F, al-Hamdan Y, Baldauf C, Gisclon L, Wesnes K, Curtin CR, Stubbs CR, Walker SA, Brunner-Ferber F. Incremental dosage of the new antipsychotic mazapertine induces tolerance to cardiovascular and cognitive effects in healthy men. *Clin Pharmacol Ther* 1996; **59**(6): 675–685.

Kongsamut S, Roehr JE, Cai J, Hartman HB, Weissensee P, Kerman LL, Tang L, Sandrasagra A. Iloperidone binding to human and rat dopamine and 5-HT receptors. *Eur J Pharmacol* 1996; **317**: 417–423.

Lesko LJ, Williams RL. Regulatory perspective: the role of pharmacokinetics and pharmacodynamics. In: Cutler NR, Sramek JJ, Narang PK eds.

Pharmacodynamics and Drug Development: Perspectives in Clinical Pharmacology. Chichester: John Wiley & Sons, 1994, p. 115–130.

Lucas RA, Heaton J, Carter GV, Satterwhite JH. Single and multiple-dose safety, pharmacodynamics, and pharmacokinetics of xanomeline, a novel muscarinic M_1 agonist, in healthy male subjects. Presented at the *Alzheimer's and Parkinson's Diseases Recent Developments, Third International Conference,* Chicago, IL, November, 1993.

Medina A, Bodick N, Goldberger AL, MacMahon M, Lipsitz LA. Effects of central muscarinic-1 receptor stimulation on blood pressure regulation. *Hypertension* 1997; **29**(3): 828–834.

Meltzer LT, Christoffersen CL, Corbin AE, Ninteman FW, Serpa KA, Wiley JN, Wise LD, Heffner TG. CI-1007, a dopamine partial agonist and potential antipsychotic agent. II. Neurophysiological and behavioral effects. *J Pharmacol Exp Ther* 1995; **274**(2): 912–920.

Miller AL, Maas JW, Contreras S, Seleshi E, True JE, Bowden C, Castiglioni J. Acute effects of neuroleptics on unmedicated schizophrenic patients and controls. *Biol Psychiatry* 1993; **34**: 178–187.

Oberholzer AF, Hendriksen C, Monsch AU, Heirli B, Stahelin HB. Safety and effectiveness of low-dose clozapine in psychogeriatric patients: a preliminary study. *Int Psychiogeriatr* 1992; **4**(2): 187–195.

Okuma, T. Differential sensitivity to the effects of psychotropic drugs: psychotics vs normals; Asian vs Western populations. *Folia Psychiatrica et Neurologica Japonica* 1981; **35**: 79–87.

Owen F, Cross AF, Crow TJ, Longden A, Poulter M, Riley GJ. Increased dopamine receptor sensitivity in schizophrenia. *Lancet* 1978; **2**: 223–226.

Padich RA, McCloskey TC, Kehne JH. 5-HT modulation of auditory and visual sensorimotor gating: II. Effects of the $5\text{-}HT_{2A}$ antagonist MDL 100,907 on disruption of sound and light prepulse inhibition produced by 5-HT agonists in Wistar rats. *Psychopharmacology (Berl)* 1996; **124**(1–2): 107–116.

Peck CC, Barr WH, Benet LZ, Collins J, et al. Opportunities for integration of pharmacokinetics, pharmacodynamics, and toxicokinetics in rational drug development. *J Clin Pharmacol* 1994; **34**: 111–119.

Physician's Desk Reference, 51st edition. Montvale, NJ: Medical Economics Data, 1997.

Pokorny R, Finkel MJ, Robinson WT. Normal volunteers should not be used for bioavailability or bioequivalence studies in clozapine. *Pharm Res* 1994; **11**(8): 1221.

Psychopharmacologic Drugs Advisory Committee. Meeting on buspirone, Bethesda, MD, September, 1983.

Puri SK, Ho I, Hsu R, Lassman HB. Multiple-dose pharmacokinetics, safety, and tolerance of velnacrine (HP 029) in healthy elderly subjects: a potential therapeutic agent for Alzheimer's disease. *J Clin Pharmacol* 1990; **30**(10): 948–955.

Puri SK, Hsu R, Ho I, Lassman HB. Single dose safety, tolerance, and pharmacokinetics of HP 029 in young men: a potential Alzheimer's agent. *J Clin Pharmacol* 1989; **29**: 278–284.

Puri SK, Hsu RS, Ho I, Lassman HB. Singe dos safety, tolerance, and pharmacokinetics of HP 029 in healthy elderly men: a potential Alzheimer's agent. *Curr Ther Res* 1988; **44**: 766–780.

Ranjan R, Meltzer HY. Acute and long-term effectiveness of clozapine in treatment-resistant psychotic depression. *Biol Psychiatry* 1996; **40**: 253–258.

Reece PA, Bockbrader H, Sedman AJ. Safety, pharmacodynamics, and pharmacokinetics of a new muscarinic agonist, CI-979. *Clin Exp Pharmacol Physiol* 1992; **21**(Suppl): 58.

Riekkinen P Jr, Schmidt B, Riekkinen M. Behavioral characterization of metrifonate-improved acquisition of spatial information in medial septum-lesioned rats. *Eur J Pharmacol* 1997; **323**(1): 11–19.

Rugsley TA, Davis MD, Akunne HC, Cooke LW, Whetzel SZ, MacKenzie RG, Shih YH, van Leeuwen DH, DeMattos SB, Georgic LM, et al. CI-1007, a dopamine partial agonist and potential antipsychotic agent. I. Neurochemical effects. *J Pharmacol Exp Ther* 1995; **274**(2): 898–911.

Schwartz JT, Brotman AW. A clinical guide to antipsychotic drugs. *Drugs* 1992; **44**(6): 981–992.

Scott JA, Crews FT. Rapid decrease in rat brain beta adrenergic receptor binding during combined antidepressant alpha-2 antagonist treatment. *J Pharmacol Exp Ther* 1983; **224**: 640–646.

Shannon HE, Bymaster FP, Calligaro DO, Greenwood B, Mitch CH, Sawyer BD, Ward JS, Wong DT, Olesen PH, Sheardown MJ, et al. Xanomeline: a novel muscarinic receptor agonist with functional selectivity for M1 receptors. *J Pharmacol Exp Ther* 1994; **269**(1): 271–281.

Sramek JJ, Anand R, Wardle TS, Irwin P, Hartman RD, Cutler NR. Safety/tolerability trial of SDZ ENA 713 in patients with probable Alzheimer's disease. *Life Sci* 1996b; **58**(15): 1201–1207.

Sramek JJ, Block GA, Reines SA, Sawin SF, Barchowsky A, Cutler NR. A multiple-dose safety trial of eptastigmine in Alzheimer's disease, with pharmacodynamic observations of red blood cell cholinesterase. *Life Sci* 1995a; **56**(5): 319–326.

Sramek JJ, Cutler NR, Kurtz NM, Murphy MF, Carta A. *Optimizing the Development of Antipsychotic Drugs*. Chichester, England: John Wiley & Sons, 1997.

Sramek JJ, Eldon MA, Posvar EL, Feng MR, Jhee SS, Hourani J, Sedman AJ, Cutler NR. Initial safety, tolerability, pharmacodynamics and pharmacokinetics of CI-1007 in patients with schizophrenia. *Psychopharm Bull*, in press.

Sramek JJ, Fresquet A, Marion-Landais G, Hourani J, Jhee SS, Martinez L, Jensen CM, Bolles K, Carrington AT, Cutler NR. Establishing the maximum tolerated dose of lesopitron in patients with generalized anxiety disorder: a bridging study. *J Clin Psychopharmacol* 1996a; **16**(6): 454–458.

Sramek JJ, Hurley DJ, Wardle TS, Satterwhite JH, Hourani J, Dies F, Cutler, NR. The safety and tolerance of xanomeline tartrate in patients with Alzheimer's disease. *J Clin Pharmacol* 1995c; **35**(8): 800–806.

Sramek JJ, Jasinsky O, Chang S, Shu V, Kashkin K, Kennedy S, Sadd C, Cutler NR. Pilot efficacy trial of ABT-200 in patients with major depressive disorder. *Depression* 1994/1995; **2**: 315–318.

Sramek JJ, Sedman AJ, Reece PA, Hourani J, Bockbrader H, Cutler NR. Safety and tolerability of CI-979 in patients with Alzheimer's disease. *Life Sci* 1995b; **57**(5): 503–510.

Strupczewski JT, Bordeau KJ, Chiang Y, Glamkowski EJ, Conway PG, Corbett R, Hartman HB, Szewczak MR, Wilmot CA, Helsley GC. 3-[(Aryloxy) alkyl] piperidinyl]-1,2-benzisoxazoles as D2/5-HT2 antagonists with potential antipsychotic activity: antipsychotic profile of iloperidone (HP873). *J Med Chem* 1995; **38**(7): 1119–1131.

Szewczak MR, Corbett R, Rush DK, Wilmot CA, Conway PG, Strupczewski JT, Cornfeldt M. The pharmacological profile of iloperidone, a novel atypical antipsychotic agent. *J Pharmacol Exp Ther* 1995; **274**(3): 1404–1413.

Unni LK, Womack C, Hannant ME, Becker RE. Pharmacokinetics and pharmacodynamics of metrifonate in humans. *Methods Find Exp Clin Pharmacol* 1994; **16**(4): 285–289.

van Kamman DP, McEvoy JP, Targum SD, Kardatzke D, Sebree TB. A randomized, controlled, dose-ranging trial of sertindole in patients with schizophrenia. *Psychopharmacology (Berl)* 1996; **124**(1–2): 168–175.

Weissman L. Multiple-dose phase I trials—normal volunteers or patients? One viewpoint. *J Clin Pharmacol* 1981; **21**(10): 385–387.

Williams RL. Dosage regimen design: pharmacodynamic considerations. *J Clin Pharmacol* 1992; **32**: 597–602.

Zelle RE, Hancock AA, Buckner SA, Basha FZ, Tietje K, DeBernardis JF, Meyer MD. Synthesis and pharmacological characterization of ABT-200: a putative novel antidepressant combining potent α-2 antagonism with moderate NE uptake inhibition. *Bioorg Med Chem Lett* 1994; **4**: 1319–1322.

Zimbroff DL, Kane JM, Tamminga CA, Daniel DG, Mack RJ, Wozniak PJ, Sebree TB, Wallin BA, Kashkin KB. Controlled, dose-response study of sertindole and haloperidol in the treatment of schizophrenia: sertindole study group. *Am J Psychiatry* 1997; **154**(6): 782–791.

6 Regulatory issues

The FDA is charged with the daunting task of ensuring that consumers in the United States are provided with safe and effective therapies. To achieve this goal, regulators must evaluate a drug development program using the highest scientific standards possible. In recent years, however, pressure has been building to complete these rigorous evaluations in a more timely fashion. To this end, the FDA has taken several measures to streamline the drug development process and to accelerate drug review and approval, many of which will be discussed in this chapter.

Efforts to speed drug development and approval appear to be successful at this time. Although the FDA is considered to have some of the most demanding regulatory requirements in the world, evidence indicates that the United States is also a world leader in drug approval. A recent study comparing the marketing approval dates of 214 new drugs introduced onto the world market from January 1990 to December 1994 showed that the United States had a similar pattern of drug availability as the United Kingdom, outpacing both Germany and Japan for 'global drugs' ultimately approved in more than one country (Kessler et al., 1996). When compared to any of the other three countries included in the analysis, patients in the United States were shown to have greater access to the majority of 'priority' drugs and to be spared at least two products that later proved to be ineffective or to cause serious adverse events.

Moreover, in a continuing effort to optimize the drug development process, regulatory agencies in the United States, the European Union, and Japan have joined together with industry representatives to promote the international harmonization of regulatory requirements through The International Conference of Harmonization of Technical Requirements for the Registration of Pharmaceuticals for Human Use (ICH). ICH is made up of six sponsors, including the FDA's Centers for Drug Evaluation and Research and Biologics Evaluation and Research, the European Commission, the European Federation of Pharmaceutical Industries

Associations, the Japanese Ministry of Health and Welfare, and the Japanese Pharmaceutical Manufacturers Association.

ICH was formed in order to pursue scientifically based and internationally harmonized technical procedures for pharmaceutical development. The industry guidelines prepared under the auspices of ICH thus reflect the FDA's current thoughts on various aspects of drug development, and can provide a convenient and up-to-date perspective on specific topics currently under consideration. With regulatory agencies around the world participating in efforts to streamline and optimize the drug development process, many issues have been raised which will need to be resolved as the pharmaceutical industry moves into the 21st century.

ARE TWO OR MORE PIVOTAL STUDIES NECESSARY?

The FDA generally requires at least two adequate and well-controlled studies to provide evidence of drug efficacy. However, the FDA has begun to explore several initiatives aimed at accelerating development, including more flexible trial designs and the potential for approval based on a single study.

One approach to expediting the development process is the 'large, simple trial.' These studies would employ relaxed inclusion and exclusion criteria, in order to allow the enrollment of large numbers of patients. Additionally, less extensive baseline and outcome data would be collected than in traditional clinical trials. Thus, a more general patient population would be assessed, and the trials could be completed relatively quickly (Kessler and Feiden, 1995). One example of a large, simple trial is the International Study of Infarct Survival (ISIS), a placebo-controlled trial in which the safety and efficacy of an intravenous beta-blocker was evaluated in 16,000 patients in 10 countries (International Study of Infarct Survival Collaborative Group, 1986). In this study, investigators noted a 15% reduction in mortality after seven days of treatment, an effect that had not been observed in previous, smaller studies. This trial required relatively limited data collection, but its sheer size allowed investigators to detect this small, but clinically significant, effect.

Large, simple trials tend to be most feasible when the toxicity profile and mechanism of action of the investigational compound are well-characterized (Kessler and Feiden, 1995). Studies of this type allow the detection of effects of moderate size which may be masked in smaller studies. Additionally, they can provide information that will be useful in the clinical use of the drug after marketing, as the population is more diverse than in traditional trials. However, large, simple trials are not appropriate for all kinds of compounds or patient populations. For example, many CNS compounds do not have a well-characterized mechanism of action. Additionally, the target patient population can be quite heterogeneous, which could result in a difficult data analysis. Thus, the feasibility of gaining approval with this type of trial is entirely dependent upon the type of compound under investigation.

For indications where more than one type of therapy is used, factorial designs are emerging as a faster way to gather information on the effects of multiple interventions (Kessler and Feiden, 1995). The basic factorial study design includes one group of patients that receives therapy A, one that receives therapy B, one that receives both A and B, and one that receives a placebo control. In this way, the factorial design combines testing that would normally require two separate trials. This type of study has obvious applications for antiviral agents, which are often administered concurrently in the treatment of AIDS. The disadvantage of this type of design is the potential difficulty of data interpretation, if the various therapies interact in a complex manner. However, a large sample size and careful planning of statistical analysis could address such difficulties (Kessler and Feiden, 1995).

Under special circumstances, the FDA may approve a new drug based on the results of a single, traditional clinical trial. Such circumstances include situations in which a trial produces particularly compelling evidence of drug effects on survival or serious morbidity (Kessler and Feiden, 1995). For example, in the initial double-blind, multicenter, placebo-controlled study of zidovudine in AIDS, 16 patients on placebo died while only one death was observed among patients receiving active drug. The drug was thus approved on the basis of this single trial. Another example is the approval of Interferon beta-1b (Betaseron) for the treatment of multiple sclerosis. The approval of this compound was based on a single clinical trial involving 372 patients, which indicated that the admin-istration of Betaseron decreased the frequency of symptom flare-ups and kept more patients free of flare-ups over the two-year treatment period. If approvals based on a single study are found to be successful (and do not compromise patient safety), this practice could have implications for compounds meant to treat serious CNS disorders, such as severe depression, Alzheimer's disease, or schizophrenia.

FDA ACCELERATED APPROVAL: REGULATION SUBPART H

In response to public concern regarding the length of time necessary to develop and evaluate new drugs for serious or life-threatening diseases, the FDA has established several means of accelerating access to such therapies. The Treatment Investigational New Drug (IND) regulations, instituted in 1987, were instrumental in allowing the distribution of promising experimental drugs for serious illnesses on the basis of considerably less data than that required for full marketing approval. Several classes of investigational compounds have since been granted Treatment IND status, including drugs for the treatment of Alzheimer's disease, severe Parkinson's disease, severe obsessive compulsive disorder, AIDS, cancer, and other serious illnesses (Flieger, 1995). In response to the AIDS epidemic, 'parallel track' regulations issued in 1992 have allowed AIDS patients who do not qualify for clinical trials to receive experimental therapies *prior* to approval, provided that the drug is deemed to be 'promising' in preliminary studies.

More recently, Subpart H of the 21 Code of Federal Regulations (Chapter 1, Part 314) entitled 'Accelerated Approval of New Drugs for Serious or Life-Threatening Illness,' has specified two circumstances in which approval can be accelerated. First, approval can be granted on the basis of adequate and well-controlled clinical trials utilizing a surrogate endpoint that is reasonably likely to be valid. Surrogate endpoints are specifically allowed in lieu of long-term clinical endpoints such as survival or irreversible morbidity. With this type of approval, the sponsor is required to conduct further controlled trials to verify the clinical benefit of the compound after the drug is marketed (generally, these trials will already be underway). In the event that post-marketing studies fail to verify the clinical benefit of the compound, the FDA can order the drug to be removed from the market quickly.

Secondly, accelerated approval can be subject to the restricted use of the new drug once it is marketed. The FDA can institute post-marketing restrictions to limit distribution of the new drug to only certain facilities or physicians with special training or experience. Additionally, restrictions might require that specific medical procedures (e.g., blood monitoring) be performed if they are deemed essential to the safe and effective use of the new drug.

So far, the accelerated approval system appears to be working. The most dramatic evidence of this is seen in the approval times for priority drugs. The United States approved the first major antiviral compound for the treatment of HIV at the same time as the UK, and approved seven others far ahead of any other country in the world (Kessler et al., 1996). Moreover, approval times for nucleoside analogs have averaged less than six months. The implications of successful accelerated approval for the development of CNS drugs, however, are not yet clear. The difficulty of developing valid and reliable surrogate endpoints for CNS indications (reviewed in Chapter 3) may be an obstacle in gaining accelerated approval under Subpart H. However, the continuing efforts of the FDA to accelerate the review and approval of drugs for serious illnesses bodes well for the future of CNS drug development.

LONG-TERM CARCINOGENICITY TRIALS: ARE THEY TRULY NECESSARY?

Carcinogenicity studies are designed to identify the tumorigenic potential of new drugs in animals and to assess the relevant risk to humans (Guideline for Industry, 1996). The need to conduct such studies is often based on concerns raised by laboratory investigations, animal toxicology studies, or data in humans. Currently, genotoxicity studies, toxicokinetics, and mechanistic studies can be routinely performed in the preclinical safety assessment of a new drug; results of such investigations are important in the decision to perform carcinogenicity studies.

However, as carcinogenicity studies are time consuming as well as resource intensive, ICH guidelines specify that they should only be performed when human exposure warrants the need for long-term (usually 2 years) information in animals. The requirement for these studies was originally instituted for those drugs that were expected to be taken regularly by patients for a substantial part of their lifetime. The FDA has more recently specified that pharmaceuticals intended to be used for three months or more necessitate long-term carcinogenicity studies. Other countries, such as Japan, have set the duration at six months. ICH guidelines (Guideline for Industry, 1996) have agreed with the six month period, based on the assumption that most pharmaceuticals administered for a duration of three months would also be used for six months. Thus, the guidelines state that long-term carcinogenicity studies should be performed for any pharmaceutical product whose expected clinical use is continuous for at least six months. In the case of compounds for chronic or recurrent conditions which, while they may not be used continuously for six months, will be used intermittently for a significant period of time (e.g. antidepressants and anxiolytics), carcinogenicity studies are also generally considered to be necessary.

Long-term carcinogenicity studies are especially indicated if there is some cause for concern about their carcinogenic potential. Criteria for such concern, as specified by ICH guidelines (Guideline for Industry, 1996), include the following: 1) previous demonstration of carcinogenic potential within the drug class that is considered relevant to humans; 2) structure-activity relationship that suggests carcinogenic risk; 3) evidence of preneoplastic lesions in repeated-dose toxicity studies; and/or 4) long-term tissue retention of parent compound or metabolite(s), resulting in local tissue reactions or other pathophysiological responses. These criteria are considered to be the most important reasons to conduct carcinogenicity studies for most categories of drugs.

Another situation in which long-term carcinogenicity studies may be warranted is where drugs are shown to significantly increase levels of endogenous peptides or proteins, such as hormones. This factor may be of particular concern with antipsychotic drugs, many of which increase levels of prolactin and/or growth hormone.

For example, concerns were raised when development of the antipsychotic risperidone revealed that its D_2 receptor antagonist activity resulted in significant elevations of prolactin in rodents and humans. Drugs with this mechanism of action are commonly associated with an increase in endocrine tumors in rodent carcinogenicity bioassays (specifically, mammary gland, pituitary, and endocrine pancreatic tumors). Thus, following the approval meeting of risperidone, the Psychopharmacologic Drugs Advisory Committee also held a special meeting to discuss the preclinical toxicity relevant to the risk/benefit ratio of risperidone. Of major concern were the results of a two-year carcinogenicity study which indicated that male rats on risperidone demonstrated a significant increase in mammary gland carcinomas, an effect that is unique among antipsychotic compounds.

However, major differences in the hormonal and reproductive physiology between rodents and humans (including the role of prolactin) have previously been noted by the FDA's Toxicology Advisory Committee. Additionally, an epidemiological study of women who reported to a breast clinic suggested that prolactin does not increase the risk of breast cancer. Finally, other drugs which stimulate the release of prolactin, such as reserpine and methyldopa, have not been associated with an increase in breast cancer. Thus, in this case, it was concluded that the relevance of rodent endocrine tumors to human risk is unknown at this time, and the safety concerns associated with elevated prolactin could be adequately addressed in risperidone's package label.

Although it is usually not considered necessary to complete long-term carcinogenicity studies prior to large-scale clinical trials, they generally must be completed prior to marketing approval. Exceptions include drugs meant to treat life-threatening or severely debilitating diseases, especially where no standard alternative therapies exist. Additionally, in cases where the life expectancy of the intended population is short (i.e., less that 2–3 years), there are usually no requirements for long-term carcinogenicity studies. These exceptions do not generally encompass drugs for CNS indications.

Currently, regulatory requirements suggest that long-term carcinogenicity studies be conducted in two rodent species, usually the rat and the mouse. There has been some question regarding the necessity of testing two separate species, and the potential savings in time and resources that could be achieved by streamlining the process to include only one. Of course, the principal issue is whether testing in one species is sufficient to assess the relevant carcinogenic risk of a new drug to humans. The rationale for conducting long-term studies in two species is the identification of trans-species tumorigens which are considered to pose a relatively higher risk to humans that single-species tumorigens. Additionally, there has been some question as to whether all studies need to be long-term. Several alternative experimental animal models are currently under investigation which could prove useful in the assessment of carcinogenicity. One alternative program that the FDA has considered includes one long-term rodent carcinogenicity study, supplemented by one additional in vivo carcinogenicity study (Federal Register, 1996; Contrera et al., 1997). This additional in vivo study can involve a short or medium-term test system, including rodent initiation-promotion models, transgenic rodent models, or newborn rodent models. To aid the interpretation of these results, mechanistic studies have also been recommended, to provide a perspective on the relevance of the data to human risk. These studies can include the examination of cellular changes (morphology, histochemistry, function), biochemical measures (dose dependence of hormone elevations), or additional genotoxicity tests (tumor induction in target organs).

HOW MANY YEARS OF HUMAN EXPOSURE ARE REQUIRED?

Pre-marketing clinical trials are expected to provide a reasonable safety profile of the compound under investigation. For drugs which are intended for acute use, the characterization of short-term safety can be achieved relatively easily with traditional trials lasting weeks to months. Drugs which are intended for chronic or repeated intermittent use, however, may require the assessment of a longer duration of exposure in order to characterize potential adverse events. Most CNS compounds fall into this latter category.

Available evidence suggests that most adverse events first occur (and are most frequent) within the first few months of drug treatment (Guideline for Industry, 1995). Thus, ICH guidelines suggest that a group of patients treated for six months (at doses that are intended for clinical use) should be adequate to assess the adverse event profile over time. Of course, this cohort of patients should be large enough to allow the assessment of whether more frequently occurring adverse events increase of decrease over time, and the observation of delayed adverse events of reasonable frequency (i.e., approximately 0.5–5%). In general, 300–600 patients should be acceptable (Guideline for Industry, 1995).

However, with drugs intended for chronic use, there is some concern that adverse events could increase in frequency or severity over time, or that serious adverse events could occur after a drug has been administered for more than six months. Thus, regulators recommend that some patients be treated for a period of one year (Guideline for Industry, 1995). The selection of the number of patients to be followed for one year should be based on the probability of detecting a given adverse event frequency, as well as practical considerations; however, ICH guidelines have suggested that 100 patients should be acceptable in most situations. The one-year exposure data should be collected in prospective studies that include doses that are intended for clinical use. If no serious adverse events are observed in these studies, then the database of 100 patients provides reasonable assurance that the true cumulative one-year incidence is no greater than 3% (Guideline for Industry, 1995).

Of course, there are exceptions to these general guidelines. For example, if there is special concern that the investigational drug will be associated with delayed adverse events, or that adverse events will increase in frequency and severity over time, then a larger group of patients followed for a longer period of time might be warranted. Special concern could be based on data from several sources, including animal studies, clinical information from drugs of a similar pharmacological class, or pharmacodynamic properties of the compound that are associated with specific adverse events. Additionally, a larger long-term sample could be required if there is a need to quantify the occurrence rate of known, specific low-frequency adverse events. This situation could arise if a specific serious adverse event has been observed with drugs of a similar structure or class, or if a rare, serious adverse event is observed in early clinical trials. Larger long-term studies might also be indicated if there is a need to assess the risk/benefit ratio of an investigational drug that has either a small clinical effect, is beneficial in only a small fraction of treated patients, or has an uncertain level of efficacy (e.g., based on a surrogate endpoint; Guideline for Industry, 1995).

However, for many classes of drugs, the above guidelines are considered to provide adequate safety information to warrant the marketing approval of an investigational compound. Of course, extensive safety data will also be gathered after the drug is marketed, providing a means to assess very long-term effects of the compound. Additionally, the characterization of very rare adverse events is not expected in pre-marketing clinical trials, and is also the domain of post-marketing research.

ROLE OF POST-MARKETING DATA IN DRUG DEVELOPMENT

The process of drug development does not end once a drug is approved. Indeed, a great deal of important information is gathered after a drug is marketed and introduced into the general patient population. As Lasagna (1980) has noted, 'information about a drug is never complete.'

Why Do We Need Post-Marketing Data?

While randomized controlled trials are the backbone of the drug development process, post-marketing data provide complementary information about a drug that cannot be gathered in the context of pre-marketing clinical trials. Because randomized controlled trials are designed to control for patient factors which could confound safety or efficacy results, we often do not know the implications of these factors until after the drug is introduced into the general patient population. Additionally, as larger numbers of patients are exposed to the marketed drug for longer periods of time, it becomes possible to gather increasingly comprehensive safety data.

The number of individuals exposed to a new drug prior to its approval can range between several hundred and several thousand. Thus, although the general adverse event profile should be well characterized in pre-marketing clinical trials, adverse events that occur at low frequencies might not be detected. For example, an adverse event which occurs in one in 5000 or even one in 1000 users could be missed in clinical trials, but could present a significant safety risk in the general market (Kessler, 1993). If an event, such as rare blood dyscrasia, occurs in 1 in 1000 treated patients, then a rough rule of thumb would require 3000 treated patients in order to provide the confidence of having the event present itself for detection at least once in the treated sample population.   One notable example of such an effect is agranulocytosis in patients treated with clozapine. Here, a genetic or other susceptibility lead to a number of deaths in Finland in the early 1970's. This unfortunate event might not have been detected in even a very large drug development program conducted in a non-susceptible population.   Furthermore, practical constraints often limit the duration of clinical trials to weeks or months, while in actual practice, many drugs will be taken intermittently or regularly for a period of years. Adverse events that develop on a very long-term basis, or with chronic exposure, are therefore also likely to go undetected.

In the case of nomifensine, an antidepressant that had been available in Germany since 1976, the compound had been prescribed to approximately 10 million patients prior to its marketing in the United States in 1985. At the time of its approval in the United States, the FDA was aware of less than 20 cases of hemolytic anemia, all non-fatal. However, in 1985, reports suggesting that hemolytic anemia could be fatal resulted in a changes to the product label to reflect this potential danger. An increase in the number of serious hemolytic anemia cases in Europe eventually caused the manufacturer to announce the withdrawal of the drug from worldwide markets in 1986. This case illustrates how the safety profile of a compound continues to develop even after marketing, and how even after 10 years of experience, new information can be discovered which will substantially impact the clinical use of a drug.

The stringent inclusion and exclusion criteria employed at the pre-marketing stage are necessary to reduce variability and increase the power of the statistical analysis; however, the resulting patient homogeneity may mean that the sample is not representative of the broader population that will be using the drug after approval. For example, many clinical protocols restrict patient age, resulting in an under-representation of both the very young and very old. Thus, the optimal doses selected at the pre-marketing stage could be inaccurate for these populations, due to potential metabolic differences. Females also tend to be under-represented in clinical trials, and there is some indication that gender-based pharmacokinetic differences exist. Pregnant or nursing females are almost universally excluded due to the risk of teratogenic and mutagenic effects, resulting in inadequate data on a drug's safety during and after pregnancy.

With any newly marketed compound, drug interaction effects are an important unknown factor. Pre-marketing clinical trials generally do not explore all potential drug interaction effects, as patients are carefully screened for concomitant medications. This factor can be of particular concern with drugs for elderly patients, such as Alzheimer's disease compounds, since most elderly patients are more likely to have a regimen including several types of drugs (Stewart and Cooper, 1994). Similarly, patients with concomitant diseases are also generally excluded from clinical trials; thus, the effect of comorbid conditions cannot be fully evaluated prior to marketing.

The treatment setting can also be a significant factor in drug safety and efficacy. For example, clozapine is a beneficial drug when close patient monitoring is possible, but can present a significant risk if regular blood count evaluations are not performed (Linden, 1993). Additionally, as patient compliance tends to be high in the clinical trial setting due to extensive monitoring, drug performance could be affected under conditions of less optimal compliance.

Although clinical trials of a new drug narrowly define the intended indication, widely marketed drugs may be provided for patients with other conditions by physicians (who should inform the patients that they are receiving the drug for a non-FDA approved indication). However, the use of a drug for any condition other than those specified in the labeling may significantly affect the risk-to-benefit ratio. Thus, the safety profile of the compound in so called 'off-label' indications can also be evaluated through post-marketing research. In many cases, the new drug could gain approval for expanded indications after post-marketing studies are completed.

Methods in Post-marketing Research

Post-marketing surveillance encompasses a number of pharmaco-epidemiological techniques that are used to gather information once a drug is approved and marketed. In the United States, the primary tool in this area is MEDWatch: The FDA Medical Products Reporting Program, which was introduced in 1993 to streamline and improve the reporting process. This program utilizes a computerized database, which includes individual spontaneous reports of certain adverse events believed to be associated with the administration of marketed drugs. The system relies on the vigilance and observation of practicing health care providers and consumers to identify and report such adverse events.

The MEDWatch system does not require that there be an established connection between the adverse event and the marketed drug. Only a *suspicion* that a relationship exists is necessary. Of course, not all adverse events are of interest in post-marketing surveillance; to report every reaction would overwhelm the system and would not be of practical use to the FDA. Thus, the FDA is particularly interested in serious adverse events, defined as responses that are fatal or life-threatening, permanently disabling, require inpatient hospitalization, or that involve congenital abnormalities, cancer, or overdose; serious and other types of adverse events associated with drugs in the first three years of marketing; and product quality defects or mislabeling. These reports are submitted either directly to the FDA or the manufacturer of the product, who is required by regulation to forward all such reports to the FDA. Indeed, the majority of cases in the FDA database are contributed by manufacturing companies (Johnson and Tanner, 1993). The information provided by MEDWatch is then used to identify potential warning signs of safety concerns.

Other databases are also available to the FDA, including the World Health Organization's adverse drug experience database, which is located in Uppsala, Sweden. Reports submitted to the FDA are also fed into WHO's database, which, along with information generated from other countries, creates an international resource of drug safety data.

Post-marketing studies provide another tool to gather additional safety information once a drug is approved. These studies can sometimes be a condition of the approval itself, if there is reason to believe that further study is necessary. Alternatively, the need to conduct such studies can arise from information gathered in spontaneous reports. Post-marketing studies can take many forms (Linden, 1993). *Randomized controlled trials* can be conducted to test for specific, suspected causal relationships and dose-response information. *Comprehensive observation studies* assess the treatment course of new drugs in a limited number of patients in the clinical setting, and are best suited to identify acute adverse events with mild to moderate severity and high incidence rates. *Phase IV intervention studies*, in contrast, target the identification of less common events. These studies are designed to answer specific questions, and require intervention into the treatment course of a limited number of patients. *Case-control studies* test for direct causal relationships, and involve a comparison of exposure rates and adverse effects of the marketed drug in cohorts of patients and defined, non-exposed controls. However, documentation of treatment and the suspected adverse event in a routine treatment must be available for these studies to be possible. *Data bank comparisons* can also be used to assess potential relationships between drug administration and specific outcomes, such as suicide in depression, or mortality rates with cancer chemotherapy.

Limitations of Post-marketing Surveillance

Spontaneous adverse event reporting and the MEDWatch system have been instrumental in identifying significant safety concerns with marketed drugs. However, there are some potential limitations as well. One of the greatest concerns is under-reporting on the part of health care providers and consumers. One study found that only approximately 1% of serious adverse events are reported to the FDA (Scott et al., 1987). A recent study conducted in France, which has a mandatory pharmacovigilance system, found that general practitioners reported only 1 out of every 4610 serious and unlabeled adverse drug reactions (Moride et al., 1997). Kessler (1993) has attributed potential under-reporting to a propensity to attribute unexpected adverse events to disease course, the limited training of medical students in clinical pharmacology and therapeutics, and the fact that reporting drug-related events to the FDA is not an ingrained practice in the United States. There is also some concern that certain terms used to define serious adverse events (such as 'significant' or 'persistent' disability) could lead to some confusion over what events should be reported (Shader and Greenblatt, 1993).

Another concern, which has potentially serious implications, is liability. Shader and Greenblatt (1993) point out that many physicians are reluctant to report adverse events because of the risk of personal liability for unexpected outcomes. To this end, the FDA has voiced its commitment to maintaining the confidentiality of the patients and those reporting the adverse events (Kessler, 1993). Moreover, a regulation extending protection against disclosure by pre-empting states discovery laws regarding voluntary reports held by pharmaceutical, biological, or medical device manufacturers was instituted in 1995.

Despite any limitations, the MEDWatch system has been quite successful in identifying rare and serious adverse events associated with new drugs. However, detecting rare adverse events is only one aspect of post-marketing research. There are many other questions (Box 6.1) which could contribute significantly to optimal clinical use, but are not generally addressed in Phase IV (Lasagna, 1980). Thus, post-marketing research is an area open to innovative methods, which could expand the scope of this already vital aspect of drug development.

BOX 6.1 ADDITIONAL QUESTIONS FOR POST-MARKETING RESEARCH

Are physicians using the drug for the labeled indication(s)? If not, why?
Is the drug performing as expected?
Is the adverse event profile as predicted from clinical trials?
Is abuse of the drug a problem?
Have new uses of the drug been noted?

Adapted from Lasagna (1980)

Future Directions

For several years, there have been discussions regarding the expanded role of post-marketing studies in drug development. Specifically, more formal programs of studying drugs after registration have been proposed as a means of accelerating pre-marketing drug development and approval, as a sort of trade-off that would suit the needs of manufacturers hoping to bring their new compounds to market as well as regulators who are concerned about unexpected drug toxicity (Lasagna, 1980; Kessler and Feiden, 1995; Winterer and Herrmann, 1996). In fact, a larger emphasis on post-marketing study has already been instituted for many compounds approved under the auspices of 21 CFR Subpart H, although reasonable evidence of therapeutic benefit must still be demonstrated prior to marketing.

REFERENCES

Contrera JF, Jacobs AC, DeGeorge JJ. Carcinogenicity testing and the evaluations of regulatory requirements for pharmaceuticals. *Regul Toxicol Pharmacol* 1997; **25**(2): 130–145.

Federal Register. International conference on harmonisation: draft guideline on testing for carcinogenicity of pharmaceuticals. August 21, 1996; **61**(163): 1–8.

Flieger K. FDA finds new ways to speed treatments to patients. *FDA Consumer Special Report on New Drug Development in the United States.* January, 1995.

Guideline for Industry. The extent of population exposure to assess clinical safety: for drugs intended for long-term treatment of non-life-threatening conditions. March, 1995.

Guideline for Industry. The need for long-term rodent carcinogenicity studies of pharmaceuticals. March, 1996.

International Study of Infarct Survival Collaborative Group. Randomised trial of intravenous atenolol among 16,027 cases of suspected acute myocardial infarction: ISIS-1. *Lancet* 1986; **2**(8498): 57–66.

Johnson JM, Tanner LA. Postmarketing surveillance: curriculum for the clinical pharmacologist. Part II: clinical and regulatory considerations. *J Clin Pharmacol* 1993; **33**: 1015–1022

Kessler DA. Introducing MEDWatch. A new approach to reporting medication and device adverse effects and product problems. *JAMA* 1993; **269**(21): 2765–2768.

Kessler DA, Feiden KL. Faster evaluation of vital drugs. *Scientific American* March 1995; 48–54.

Kessler DA, Hass AE, Feiden KL, Lumpkin MD, Temple R. Approval of new drugs in the United States: Comparison with the United Kingdom, Germany, and Japan. *JAMA* 1996; **276**(22): 1826–1831.

Lasagna L. Post-marketing surveillance. *Triangle* 1980; **19**(3–4): 107–111.

Linden M. Postmarketing surveillance of psychotherapeutic medications: a challenge for the 1990's. *Psychopharmacol Bull* 1993; **29**(1): 51–56.

Moride Y, Haramburu F, Requejo AA, Bégaud B. Under-reporting of adverse drug reactions in general practice. *Br J Clin Pharmacol* 1997; **43**(2): 177–181.

Scott HD, Rosenbaum SE, Waters WJ, Colt AM, Andrews LG, Juergens JP, Faich GA. Rhode Island physician's recognition and reporting of adverse drug reactions. *RI Med J* 1987; **70**(7): 311–316.

Shader RI, Greenblatt DJ. MedWatch, the new FDA adverse effects reporting system [editorial]. *J Clin Psychopharmacol* 1993; **13**(5): 303–304.

Stewart RB, Cooper JW. Polypharmacy in the aged: practical solutions. *Drugs Aging* 1994; **4**(6): 449–461.

Winterer G, Herrmann WM. Effect and efficacy – on the function of models in controlled phase III trials and the need for prospective pharmacoepidemiological studies. *Pharmacopsychiatry* 1996; **29**(4): 135–141.

7 Concluding remarks

In summary, both the pharmaceutical industry and regulatory agencies have recognized the need to accelerate drug development and approval. Continued progress in drug development is important not only for the specific drugs that are marketed, but also for the overall advances that are made in understanding disease mechanisms. However, streamlining the development process must be accomplished without compromising the high scientific standards which are necessary to ensure that only safe and effective compounds reach the marketplace.

Over the past decade, the FDA has taken an active role in streamlining drug development and approval. Innovative measures, such as approval based on surrogate endpoints or restricted use, have already helped to speed essential drugs for life-threatening or debilitating diseases to the marketplace. Careful monitoring of these compounds after marketing has also helped to ensure that patient safety is not compromised. Furthermore, increased flexibility in trial design will likely contribute to more optimal and time-efficient drug development programs in the future.

At this time, the implications of these regulatory measures for the development of CNS compounds is uncertain. While valid and reliable surrogate endpoints have remained somewhat elusive for CNS compounds, surrogate markers have already proven useful as a means to confirm a drug's central activity. In particular, biochemical or pharmacodynamic markers in CSF have provided a tool to assess a drug's central mechanism of action. The development of markers which correlate well with clinical improvement is a worthwhile endeavor, and warrants further study.

One area in which surrogate markers may play a significant role in a successful and timely drug development is proper dose selection. As discussed in Chapter 3, inaccurate or suboptimal dose selection for Phase II clinical trials can result in substantial delays or even the discontinuation of a drug development program. As the vast majority of CNS compounds have demonstrated linear dose-response curves, efficacy is sometimes observed only at the higher end of the tolerable dose range; thus, a program could be abandoned for lack of therapeutic benefit if at least the minimum effective dose is not tested. When available, CSF levels of a central surrogate marker may be the best option to guide the selection of dose ranges and intervals at an early stage in development (e.g., small, dose-finding studies in the patient population).

As differences in drug tolerance between patients and healthy subjects have been observed for a wide variety of CNS compounds, we have stressed the importance of the bridging study in early clinical development. Our experience in conducting bridging studies in indications such as Alzheimer's disease, anxiety, schizophrenia, and depression have indicated that it is quite common for patients to tolerate substantially higher, and sometimes lower, doses of CNS compounds than healthy subjects. The methodology employed in bridging studies must be tailored to the pharmacological characteristics of an individual compound, but often requires several approaches, including both fixed-dose and titration panels, in order to determine the MTD in both situations. For antipsychotic compounds which generally require titration, a titration panel to determine the maximum starting dose as well as a fixed-dose panel to determine the top dose that can be administered are recommended, along with other titration panels to find a regimen to reach the top dose quickly.

The bridging study allows the determination of the clinical dose range parameters that can be employed in Phase II/III efficacy trials. Bridging studies can optimize the dose and dosing regimen early in a development program, assisting in critical 'go/no go' decisions in Phase II. In this way, a compound can be confidently put to rest or launched into an aggressive development program relatively early in the process. The potential advantages in time savings are depicted in Figure 7.1.

Moreover, to assess central PK/PD relationships and their connection to peripheral PK/PD parameters, we have developed dynabridge methodology. A dynabridge study is a PK/PD CSF study which is conducted in the patient population. Dynabridge studies go beyond dose-finding and safety/tolerance to the evaluation of pharmacodynamic indicators of drug activity. These studies utilize a continuous CSF sampling procedure which allows the determination of central PK/PD relationships over time. CSF is analyzed for drug and metabolite concentrations, as well as for measures of drug activity (e.g. enzyme inhibition or neurotransmitter levels) while peripheral PK/PD parameters are concurrently monitored. Through the dynabridge study, the time course of drug activity across the potential dosing range is determined, allowing optimal dosing regimens to be selected prior to efficacy trials.

Accelerated development:

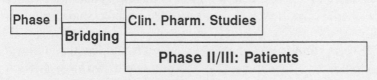

Traditional development:

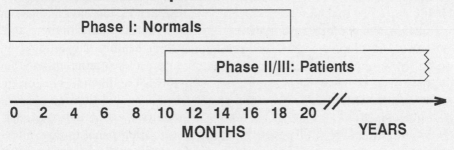

Figure 7.1 Accelerated versus traditional development timelines. Reproduced by permission from Sramek et al., 1997.

The patient population included in bridging and dynabridge studies should closely resemble that which will be enrolled in Phase II dose-ranging studies. Based on our experience of careful monitoring in these inpatient studies, the short-term safety findings are often predictive of adverse event profiles in larger trials. Ideally, bridging and dynabridge studies should lead into definitive dose-finding, placebo-controlled efficacy and safety trials.

The design of these definitive trials should take several factors into consideration, including the nature of the question under investigation, regulatory requirements, practical concerns, and ethical issues. In Chapter 4, we addressed the ethical issues involved in using placebo controls. While some have argued that the ethics of using placebos in psychotropic drug trials are questionable because patients are denied treatment with established compounds, evidence suggests that there is no substitute for the scientific control that placebo groups offer. Placebos are able to control for a variety of nonspecific effects that are potential confounding variables in the evaluation of drug efficacy, as well as to calibrate the skills of the clinical staff in a particular trial. In most cases, with careful patient selection and vigilant monitoring, we believe that placebo controls can be a safe and effective research tool.

As novel strategies for the treatment of CNS disorders arise, we must re-evaluate the appropriateness of the traditional, parallel-group design for the assessment of efficacy. This issue is particularly important for Alzheimer's disease compounds, as the focus of treatment has recently shifted from symptomatic improvement to a slowing of disease progression. Additionally, the FDA has made an effort to encourage efficient drug development strategies by increasing the range of acceptable trial designs. Novel strategies for the treatment of CNS disorders will no doubt result in innovative designs for future trials.

Drug development must be continuously evaluated and optimized in order for safer and more effective compounds to be made available to patients. We believe that bridging and dynabridge studies are important early steps which can provide a solid foundation for subsequent development. By helping to accelerate the drug development process, these studies can assure that beneficial treatments are provided for patients in a timely manner, without compromising scientific standards or safety.

Index

Index compiled by Liza Weinkove